Amal Feroui
Mohammed Amine Lazouni

Implementation of a Breast Cancer Early Detection System

Amal Feroui
Mohammed Amine Lazouni

Implementation of a Breast Cancer Early Detection System

Detection and Characterization of Mammary Masses

Imprint

Any brand names and product names mentioned in this book are subject to trademark, brand or patent protection and are trademarks or registered trademarks of their respective holders. The use of brand names, product names, common names, trade names, product descriptions etc. even without a particular marking in this work is in no way to be construed to mean that such names may be regarded as unrestricted in respect of trademark and brand protection legislation and could thus be used by anyone.

Cover image: www.ingimage.com

This book is a translation from the original published under ISBN 978-620-6-70110-1.

Publisher:
Sciencia Scripts
is a trademark of
Dodo Books Indian Ocean Ltd. and OmniScriptum S.R.L publishing group

120 High Road, East Finchley, London, N2 9ED, United Kingdom
Str. Armeneasca 28/1, office 1, Chisinau MD-2012, Republic of Moldova, Europe
Printed at: see last page
ISBN: 978-620-8-03542-6

Contents

Summary 2

GENERAL INTRODUCTION 3

Chapter 1 5

Chapter 2 17

Chapter 3 31

Bibliography 58

Summary

In this work we have implemented a system for the early detection of breast cancer, based on image processing methods in a context of aiding medical diagnosis by analysing medical imaging precisely mammography. We began with pre-processing to recover the region of interest with a cleaned background, followed by a segmentation phase to detect tumours using Watershed, region growth and K-means approaches. Finally, the segmented lesions are characterised using shape and texture attributes such as surface area, perimeter and compactness. Our approaches have been tested on the basis of "Mias" images with the implementation of an interface that can be made available to users with all possible freedom, taking advantage of the capacity of the Matlab programming language.

Key words: breast cancer, medical imaging, mammography, segmentation, LPE, region growth, K-means, MIAS, Matlab.

GENERAL INTRODUCTION

1 General introduction

Breast cancer is a major public health issue. It is a notorious cancer that threatens the lives of most women. Approximately one woman in ten is affected by this disease during her lifetime. However, reducing the mortality rate from this type of cancer and improving the chances of recovery are only possible if the tumour is treated in its earliest stages. In order to ensure early detection of such tumours, radiologists have been led to increase the frequency of mammography, particularly in the 40-50 age group. However, all radiologists recognise the difficulty of interpreting mammograms, because they represent a complex image modality to interpret, due to the variety of tissue densities, the complicated structures of the breast, and the diversity of tumours in terms of type, shape, contours, etc. The mammogram is the reference technique for breast exploration and the most effective in terms of surveillance.

Given the complexity of mammography interpretation, diagnostic assistance systems have become essential. These systems act as a 'second reader' of the image, helping the radiologist to make a diagnostic decision and pointing out possible anomalies.

The main objective of this thesis is to present some of the systems for interpreting medical images. And for the automatic enhancement and segmentation of masses in mammography images, i.e. it is a question of designing a system for recognising mammography images, the recognition is based on a segmentation of these images by a set of segmentation approaches for extracting the relevant information necessary, subsequently, in the decision procedure and classification of anomalies; while focusing on the quality of the segmentation because further processing depends closely on the result of the latter.

Outline of this report :

This project is structured around three chapters, which are presented as follows:

Chapitre1   medical context

In order to justify the algorithmic approach, it is therefore necessary first to describe the medical context of this project, which is the objective of the first chapter.

We describe the anatomy of the breast, the various benign and malignant pathologies that affect it, and then go on to describe the screening, diagnosis and treatment of cancers. We then describe general aspects of breast imaging and mammography in more detail.

Chapitre2   image processing tools

This chapter describes the various pre-processing tools, such as linear and non-linear filters and morphological filters, followed by segmentation methods: by region, contour and watershed segmentation. We end this chapter with an introduction to the characterisation and classification phase.

Chapitre3   segmentation

This chapter contains three main steps:

Stage (1): The pre-treatment stage

This is a step designed to highlight them can facilitate detection and improve image quality. And to resolve the problems of mammography artefacts.

Stage (2): The segmentation stage

This is the description of the segmentation phase after the following approaches:

- the LPE (water divide line)
- regional growth
- K-means.

Stage (3): The characterisation and production stage

In this step we extracted the characteristics of each image in order to simplify the phase. Classification and description of the development tools and the different parts of our application (implementation).

Chapter 1

Medical context

1. Introduction

Medical imaging is certainly one of the areas of medicine that has undergone a veritable revolution over the last twenty years. These recent discoveries not only enable better diagnosis, but also offer new hope for the treatment of many diseases (such as breast cancer). Breast cancer is the most common neoplasia in women worldwide, and every year around 10,000 cases of breast cancer are recorded in our country. In Algeria, this type of neoplasia is the leading malignant tumour in women, and is the leading cause of death among women, with around 3,500 deaths recorded every year. Breast cancer affects one in 11 women, most of whom are aged between 50 and 60. Only 5% of women with breast cancer are under 35. It is the most common cancer in women, and the number of cases is rising steadily. These figures show the importance of early detection of this disease. X-ray mammography remains the most reliable technique for the early diagnosis of breast cancer.

Masses and micro-calcifications are the first warning signs of this disease. The mortality rate has fallen in recent years, partly due to the use of mammography, and mass screening campaigns have been launched in most European countries. As a result of this screening, the number of mammograms to be analysed is constantly increasing, which raises the problem of the workload of specialists, who vary in their interpretation of mammograms.

Furthermore, malignant abnormalities must be detected with a high level of specificity, given the number of normal cases compared with benign cases. With this in mind, diagnostic tools have been developed to help detect lesions.

In this chapter, we look at the medical approach to breast imaging to set the context for our application.

1   Breast anatomy

The breast is a glandular organ which occupies the anterior-superior part of the thorax. The biological function of this organ is to produce milk. From an anatomical point of view, it is a mass essentially made up of fatty glandular tissue surrounded by a layer of connective tissue essential for its maintenance. At the tip of the breast is the areola, a pigmented surface containing small scattered granules, centred by the nipple, a projection into which the milk ducts open. The breast is also made up of around twenty lobules, which are glands whose role is to produce milk. Milk is transported to the nipple via the milk ducts connected to these lobules. [1]

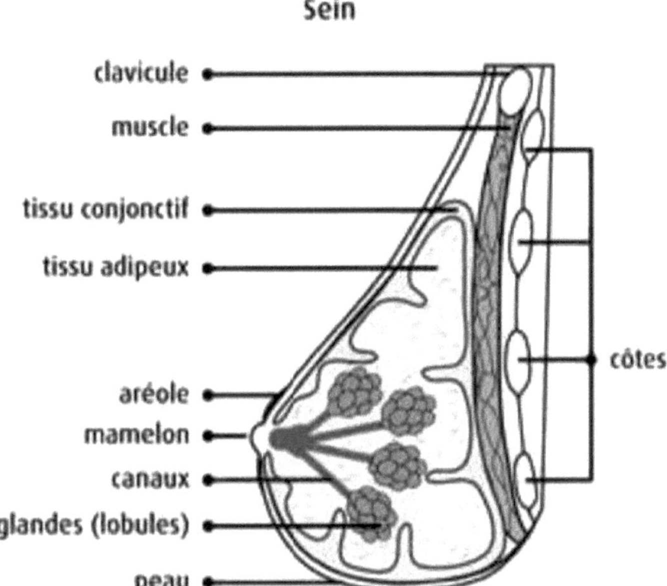

Figure 1.1: details the structure of the breast and its various components.

2 *Breast cancer*

Breast cancer is the most frequently diagnosed cancer in women worldwide. Its incidence increases with age, but it can also affect younger women, with a quarter of cases diagnosed before the age of 50. Breast cancer starts in the cells of the breast. The cancerous (malignant) tumour is a group of cancerous cells that can invade and destroy neighbouring tissue. It can also spread (metastasise) to other parts of the body. The first symptom of breast cancer is the presence of a lump in the breast, corresponding to the tumour. It may also be accompanied by hard lymph nodes in the armpit (axillary lymph nodes), indicating that the cancer has spread, as well as skin changes in the breast and nipple (padded skin and a nipple that goes in instead of out). The breast may gradually become deformed and ulcerated, sometimes resulting in discharge from the nipple on one side only. If the cancer is diagnosed late, the tumour may spread, triggering other symptoms such as nausea, vomiting, weight loss, jaundice, bone pain, headaches, shortness of breath or coughing.

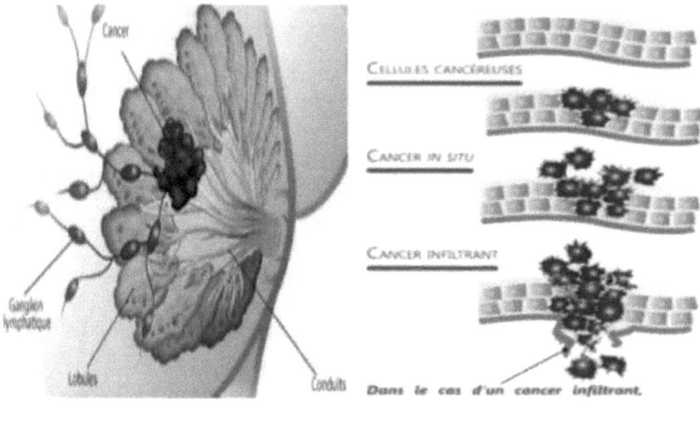

Figure 1.2 : _ a) Breast cancer. b) Types of breast cancer.

In short, breast cancer is a malignant tumour that develops from the cells that make up the mammary gland. The malignant cells multiply uncontrollably to form the tumour. When breast cancer is left untreated, the tumour cells spread locally and invade neighbouring organs. They can also spread by blood or lymph to distant organs (metastases). The organs most frequently affected by metastases are bone, lung, liver and brain. [2]

3   Breast diseases

3.1 Benign illnesses

Benign tumours have well-defined outlines. They grow slowly and remain localised in the tissue or organ in which they originate. They do not metastasise to other parts of the body. Benign tumours are composed of cells that resemble the normal cells of the tissue concerned. The most common benign tumour to develop in the breast is the fibroadenoma. Other benign breast conditions are :

Cysts, fibrocystic changes, hyperplasia, nipple discharge and gynaecomastia. Most breast masses are not benign tumours, but only a pathological examination carried out after a biopsy can verify that they are not cancerous. [3]

3.2 Malignant diseases

Malignant tumours are usually poorly defined. However, some are well defined and can be considered benign for a time, which can delay the diagnosis of cancer. The cancer cells that make up malignant tumours show various anomalies compared with normal cells: different shape and size, irregular contours, etc. They are called undifferentiated cells because they have lost their original characteristics. Malignant tumours tend to invade neighbouring tissues. They can lead to metastasis: cancerous cells escape from the primary tumour and colonise another area of the body, forming a new tumour which is called a secondary tumour or metastasis. [3]

3.3 The symptoms

The symptoms listed below do not necessarily mean that you have breast cancer. But if they do, it's important to detect it as early as possible. [4]

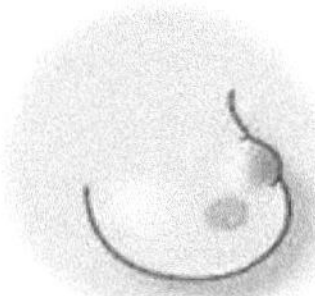

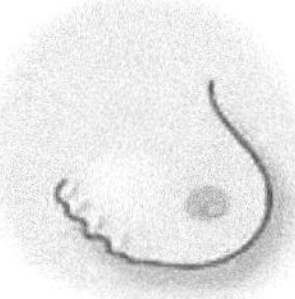

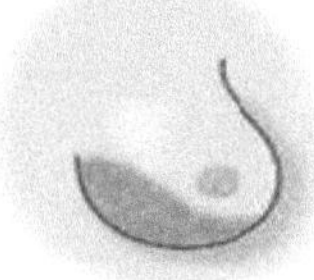

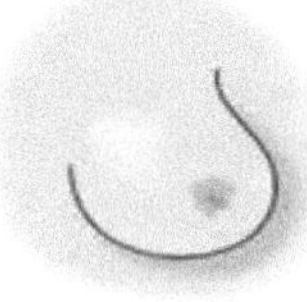

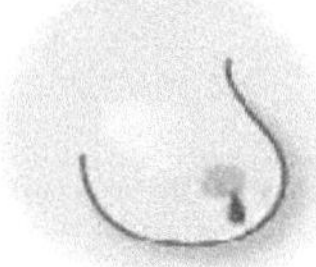

A "lump" or mass appears in the breast or under the armpit
The skin changes colour or texture
Greenish or bloody fluid coming out of the nipple

The nipple changes in appearance (e.g. it points inwards whereas before it pointed outwards)

Figure 1.3 Symptoms of breast cancer.

a)   A lump in the breast :

A lump or mass in the breast is the most common sign of breast cancer. The lump, which is generally painless, is usually hard and irregular in shape. It also appears to be "fixed" in the breast.

b)   Hard lymph nodes in the armpit:

One or more hard lumps in the armpit sometimes mean that breast cancer has spread to the axillary lymph nodes. However, the lymph nodes remain painless.

c)   Changes to the skin of the breast and nipple:

The skin of the breast may become padded (taking on the appearance of orange peel skin) or wrinkled.

d)   The nipple may point inwards, whereas it usually points outwards.

e)   The breast may become deformed and lose its shape, and wrinkles may appear.

f)   The skin of the breast may be red, scaly (ulcerated) and covered in scabs, and the skin of the nipple may start to peel.

g)   Discharge from a single nipple: can be a sign of breast cancer, particularly if it occurs without compression of the nipple and if it contains blood or is greenish.

h)   A change in the size or shape of the breast:

Redness, oedema and significant heat in the breast may be a sign of inflammatory breast cancer (inflammatory breast cancer is a rare cancer, accounting for 1 to 4% of all cases of breast cancer. Cancer cells have the characteristic of moving rapidly through the lymphatic vessels in the skin of the breast, which they eventually block. This causes local inflammation of the breast. If you notice any of these signs, you should consult your doctor immediately. The doctor will decide what further tests are necessary.

3.4 Other symptoms

If the cancer is not diagnosed as soon as the first symptoms appear, the tumour may grow and spread to other parts of the body, leading to other so-called later symptoms, such as bone pain, nausea, loss of appetite, weight loss and jaundice, shortness of breath, coughing and accumulation of fluid around the lungs (pleural effusion), headaches, double vision and muscle weakness. [4]

3.5 Screening, Diagnosis and Treatment

The incidence of breast cancer continues to rise. Various studies have confirmed that it is early detection of cancers that can improve their vital prognosis. Any change in the size or shape of the breast, changes in the skin and nipple, the presence of a hard mass with an irregular contour, as well as the presence of hard and sometimes painful lymph nodes in the armpit, requires a thorough medical examination of the breast. [5]

a) **Screening:** early **detection** of breast cancer is compulsory for women over the age of 40 every two years. The examination used is a mammogram. If an abnormality is discovered, the doctor will order additional tests (additional incidences, ultrasound, biopsy) to confirm the diagnosis of cancer.

b) **Diagnosis:** of breast cancer is based on a clinical diagnosis, mammography and pathology.

• **clinical examination**: this is an examination carried out before and after the mammogram to highlight any abnormalities in certain areas and to explain certain results. In this way, a correlation is made between clinical and imaging findings.

• **Mammography**: the essential examination for exploring the mammary gland
This may be supplemented by a breast ultrasound scan.

• **Anatomopathology**: This gives precise information about the type of breast cancer. It involves microscopic analysis of the cells and tissues removed from a breast abnormality.

c) **Treatments** can be local, systemic or both: surgery and radiotherapy act locally on cancer cells located in the breast or lymph nodes: these are local cancer treatments.

• **Surgery**: consists of removing the tumour and any cancerous grafts. There are several possible operations: breast-conserving surgery (only the tumour is removed) and total mastectomy (removal of the breast).

• **Radiotherapy:** aims to remove cancer cells using equipment that emits rays. These rays are intended to eliminate any traces of cancer that may remain after surgery.

• **Chemotherapy**: is a treatment involving the use of drugs throughout the body. The aim of these drugs is to clear the cancer cells or prevent them from growing.

• **Hormone therapy**: is a treatment that works throughout the body. Its aim is to prevent the action of certain hormones on cancer cells.

4 Medical imaging dedicated to breast cancer screening

Medical imaging is certainly one of the areas of medicine that has made the most progress over the last twenty years. These recent discoveries not only enable better diagnosis, but also offer new hope for the treatment of many diseases. Cancer, epilepsy... the precise identification of the lesion is already facilitating recourse to surgery, the only therapeutic solution for some patients. Such techniques are also helping us to better understand the workings of certain still mysterious organs, such as the breast. [6]

4.1 X-ray :

Discovered over a century ago, radiography uses X-rays, which are capable of playing tricks on matter. Passing through a certain part of the body, they print a radiographic film, which is more or less blackened depending on the organ it passes through. The "X-ray" thus resembles a Chinese shadow, with bones appearing in white and less dense structures (such as the lungs) in black. [6]

4.2 Biopsy :

It is performed using a transcutaneous needle guided by palpation or ultrasound (Fig1.10). It is carried out by a doctor, radiologist or surgeon. A sample of an abnormality is taken from the breast and sent to a pathologist for analysis to determine whether it is benign or malignant. [6]

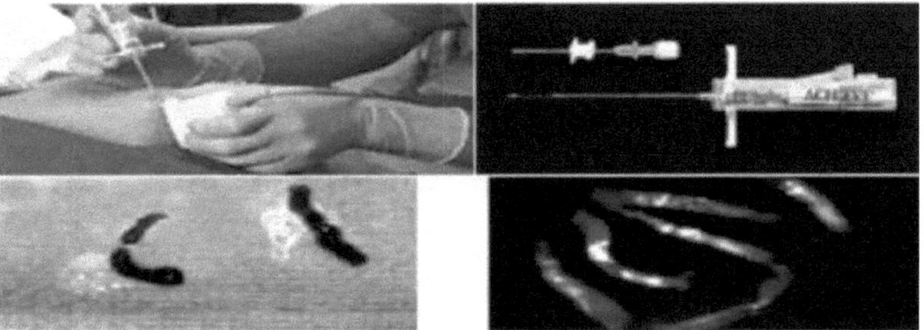

Figure 1.4 Ultrasound-guided biopsy and radiological confirmation of calcification of a sample

4.3 Ultrasound :

Ultrasound is a technique for exploring the inside of the body based on ultrasound. A probe sends a beam of ultrasound into the area of the body to be explored. Depending on the nature of the tissue, these sound waves are reflected with varying degrees of power. Processing these echoes allows the organs observed to be visualised [6].

4.4 Breast MRI :

Magnetic resonance imaging of the breast is a second-line examination that must be carried out after a full sinological work-up (clinical examination, mammography with or without ultrasound). It is much more effective in detecting infiltrating carcinomas (sensitivity ranging from 94% to 100%) than intracanal carcinomas (sensitivity varying from 77% to 94%). [6]

4.5 Breast scintigraphy :

Or lymphoscintigraphy, used in the preoperative phase to detect the location of sentinel lymph nodes, the first lymph nodes to emerge from the breast. Intraoperative analysis of these lymph nodes will reveal whether they have been invaded, which could lead to metastatic spread. [6]

4.6 PET SCAN or TEP SCAN:

(Positron Emission Tomography) is a nuclear medicine examination that can complement other radiological examinations (mammography, ultrasound, scintimammography, CT and magnetic resonance), but cannot replace them. It can sometimes be used to detect tumours in women with dense breasts, breast implants or who have undergone breast surgery. It can be used to accurately assess the spread of a cancer, and also to distinguish between a recurrence of breast cancer and changes to the breast due to surgery or radiotherapy. However, it cannot detect tumours smaller than 1 cm. [6]

4.7 Mammography
4.7.1 Definition

Mammography is an X-ray (a medical imaging technique based on the use of X-rays to see inside a part of the body) of the breasts. Mammography projects the volume of the breast onto the image plane. It enables the mammary gland to be analysed using differences in the attenuation of different types of tissue. The advantage of visualising all breast tissue in a single image is directly linked to one of its greatest shortcomings, the superimposition of different tissues traversed by the same beam and projected onto a single area of the detector. This superimposition is a source of uncertainty, since it is no longer possible to distinguish on the image between real overdensities, which correspond to a radio-opaque region in the tissue in three dimensions, and superimpositions of several tissues with relatively low densities. Mammography is somewhat unpleasant for some women because of the need to compress the breast between two plates to obtain a good quality image. [7]

4.7.2 Types of mammography

There are 2 types of mammogram:

• Screening mammography: women aged between 50 and 69 who have no signs of breast cancer have a mammogram every 2 years, as a preventive measure. This mammogram helps to detect lumps or abnormal areas of breast tissue that may be too small to be detected by hand examination of the breasts.

• Diagnostic mammography: is performed on women in whom a sign, such as a lump or abnormal breast tissue, has already been detected. This detection will have been made by the women themselves, when observing their breasts, or by a doctor during a clinical breast examination, or by a screening mammogram. The test is then more thorough and a little longer, making it possible to obtain more breast images, which are more detailed and taken from different angles than during a screening mammogram. [7]

4.7.3 Mammography equipment

The device used for mammography is the mammogram (figure 1.4). This machine consists of an X-ray tube that generates low-energy X-rays (between 20 and 50 kV) and a breast compression system. First, both breasts are compressed in turn. This compression allows the breast tissue to spread out, making it easier to visualise breast structures and reducing the dose of X-rays delivered. In the second stage, both breasts are exposed to a low dose of X-rays. This produces a projection of the breast on a flat detector. X-rays are taken using silver film or high-quality digital radiology systems. Analysis of the mammary gland is based on differences in the attenuation of different types of tissue. In the following section we detail the anatomy of the breast which subsequently allows us to establish the relationship between the nature of the breast tissue and X-ray infiltration. [7]

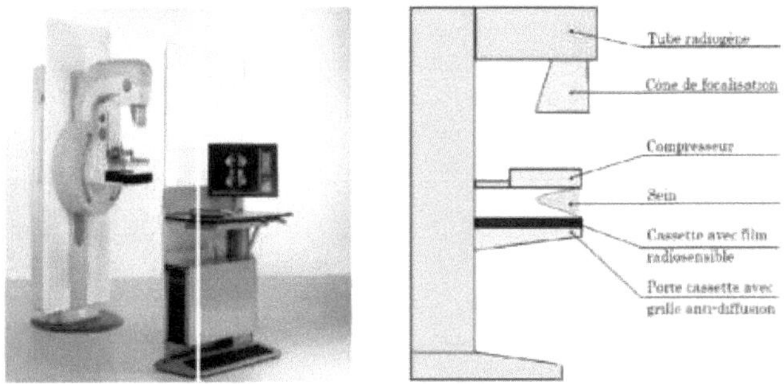

Figure 1.5 Mammography.

4.7.4 Analysis of mammography images

The mammography image is the result of the attenuation of a beam of X-rays passing through the various breast tissues. The attenuation of this beam depends essentially on the composition of the tissues passing through. [8]

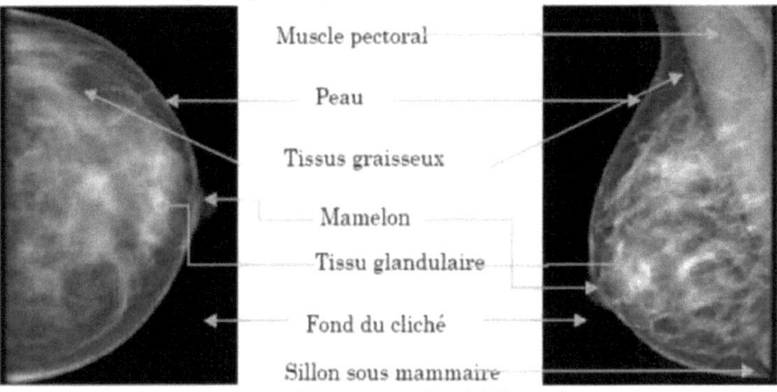

Figure 1.6 X-ray anatomy of a normal breast on a face/oblique view

4.7.5 Mammography artefacts

A digitised mammogram generally contains two distinct regions: the exposed region of the breast and the unexposed region (background). The visual interpretation of mammography often results in the identification of radio-opaque artefacts, which may be strongly related to the subject, complicating the segmentation of breast tissue and the recognition of abnormal structures.

While the human visual system can easily ignore such objects during interpretation, an automated mammography system must first identify and classify these artefacts, which cause interpretation errors during image analysis. [9]

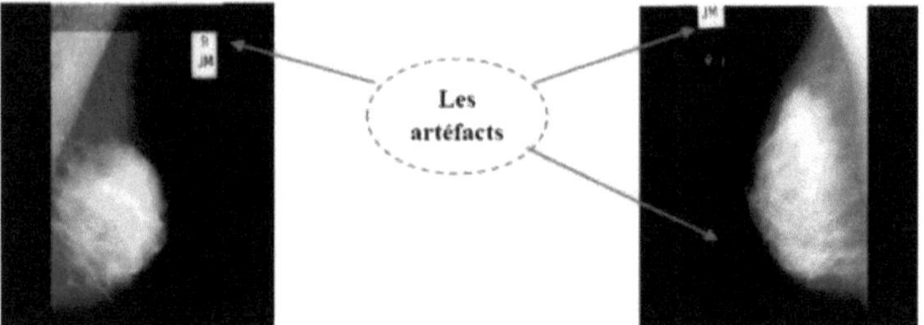

Figure 1.7: Mammography artefacts.

These artefacts fall into two main categories: film labels and opaque artefacts.

4.7.5.1 Mammography film labels :

Mammograms are generally marked with some form of permanent identification label containing information about the examination carried out. These labels are radiopaque indicators showing the laterality of the mammogram (R/L, Right/Left) as well as MLO / CC projection indicators. For example, a medio-lateral oblique (MLO) view of the right breast is marked RMLO, and a cranio-caudal (CC) view of the left breast is marked LCC [9].

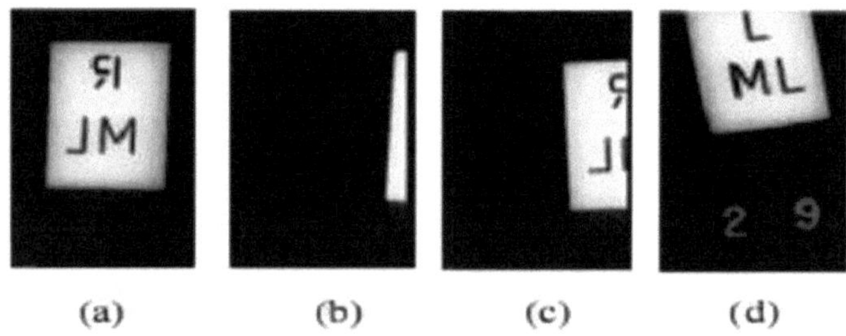

Figure 1.8: Mammography film labels: (a) full label and (b-c-d) partial labels.

4.7.5.2 Incidences in mammography

Depending on which part of the breast is being examined, different views are used. The most common views are the external oblique (or medio-lateraloblique) view and the frontal view. [9]

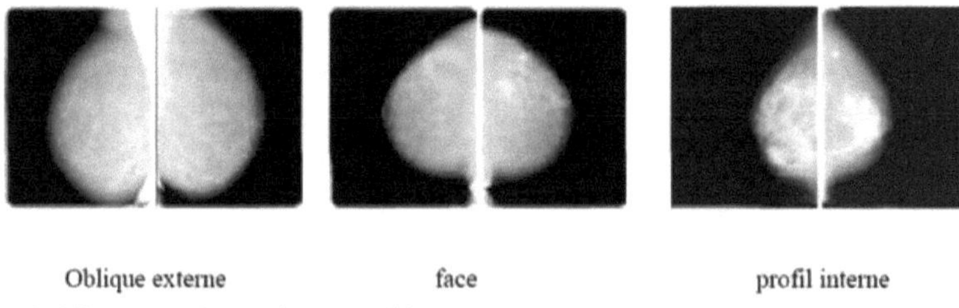

External oblique   face   inner profile

Figure 1.9: Incidence of mammography.

4.7.5.3 Radiopaque artefacts

There are two types of opaque radio artefacts: high-intensity bands or wedges and opaque markers. Opaque markers are labels where the text is in high intensity (the rectangle surrounding the text does not exist). Corners are high-intensity bands that run along the edge of the mammogram. [9]

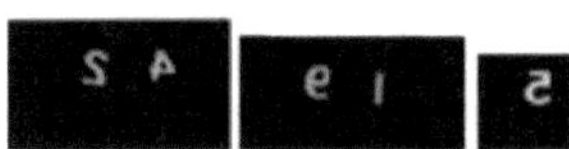 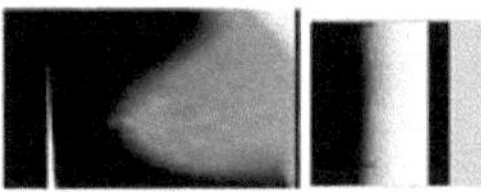

Figure 1.10: Radiopaque artefacts **Figure 1.11**: High intensity bands

4.7.6 Radiological breast anomalies

Breast cancer screening leads to the discovery of four types of purely radiological anomalies: opacities, micro-calcifications, density asymmetries and architectural distortions. This study focuses on the analysis of micro-calcifications.

* *Mammary opacities :*

An opacity is an abnormality of the connective or epithelial tissue. It corresponds to an area of abnormal overdensity, which is not distinguished from normal overdensity by a precise criterion, but by a combination of different characteristics: size, density, contour, shape, texture, etc. It will therefore be easily visible in a fatty area and much more difficult to detect in a dense area of connective tissue [10]. It is experience that enables the radiologist to distinguish an opacity on a mammogram. Over-density on several images taken at several different views is a strong presumption in favour of opacity.

* *Mammary calcifications :*

Calcifications are small calcium deposits, opaque to X-rays and visible on mammography. Their origin is not always known, but they may be linked to cellular secretions. Their morphology is determined by where they are formed. [11] A detailed analysis of calcifications reveals two main categories:

1. *macrocalcifications :*

Are coarse deposits of calcium in the breast, a very distinct appearance on mammography, They are always identified as benign conditions.

2. *microcalcifications :*

Are small calcium deposits, between (200- 500) µm, at the limit of visibility. They may be benign or malignant (Fig1.8): their nature is determined by micro- or macro-biopsy. They must be interpreted according to several criteria:

* *Size*: Calcifications in ductal cancer in situ vary greatly in size. It is the difference in size that should be taken into account when assessing calcifications.

* *Number of mcs*: As a general rule, any grouping of more than 4 calcifications should be removed when these calcifications have other features that may suggest malignancy. [11]

* *Location*: They are either diffuse, affecting a large area of the breast, or sometimes the entire ductal tree. Sometimes they are more localised. According to the work of Lanyi and Zitat, geometric formations are almost always synonymous with cancer, whereas more diffuse formations are more likely to be benign. [11]

* *Shape*: This is undoubtedly the essential element in assessing malignancy. Rounded or oval calcifications are probably the most common.

Benign. Conversely, the more irregular they are, the more likely they are to be malignant.

5 CAD (Computer-Aided Detection) system for mammography

For some years now, a number of research teams have been attempting to develop computer systems for analysing mammography images. Several avenues are being explored, including automatic classification of the anomalies detected, pattern recognition and detection. CAD computer-assisted detection systems are already on the market, and the results are widely published in the international scientific press.

A CAD is a hardware and software system that analyses medical images and assists the specialist in his detection work. More specifically, it often consists of a detector and a classifier (artificial intelligence). The detector detects microcalcifications and masses, whether benign or malignant. This gives medical significance to the detection. The

CAD does not, of course, make a diagnosis. It classifies the disease into categories: benign, malignant, normal, undetermined, etc. Some system eliminates the elements detected that are, for example, benign or normal. The rest is highlighted and left to the judgement of the doctor, who is the only one to make the diagnosis. [12]

6 Conclusion

This chapter has enabled us to highlight the value of mammography and the valuable information it provides for diagnosing tumours. The application of image processing tools enables tumours to be detected to aid and facilitate diagnosis by the doctor. To do this, we need sufficient knowledge of these tools, which is the subject of the second chapter.

Chapter 2

Mammography Image
mammography images

1   Introduction

The aim of medical image processing is to extract useful diagnostic information from the images acquired, revealing details that are difficult to see with the naked eye, while avoiding the creation of artefacts that are falsely informative. To achieve this, processing uses tools and algorithms to act on the digitised image. Shape reconstruction, segmentations, quantifications, functional analysis, even simulations (virtual organs, virtual patients), all these processing tools have contributed to improving the quality of the images acquired, to their interpretation and above all to a better approach to diagnosis.

Segmentation is one of the steps in the analysis of medical images and is considered to be an essential step in any image analysis process. It is a low-level process that precedes the measurement, understanding and decision stages. Its objective is to partition the image into related and homogeneous regions according to a homogeneity criterion.

In this chapter, we will present the various image segmentation techniques and conclude with a review of the state of the art in medical image segmentation.

2   Image processing

It is a set of operations relating to the collection, recording, processing, modification, editing, etc. of data. Let's set aside the terms recording and editing. The general principle of image processing is therefore, apart from a few details, a system that receives images, applies processing to them and produces information related to the intended application [13]. A radiation source sends waves onto an object, which are then reflected and collected by a sensor. The sensor transforms these waves into a set of points. These points are processed and information is produced at the output of the system. Image processing can be summarised in four main stages:

- *Image acquisition :*

Implementation of the physical processes involved in forming images, followed by formatting so that these images can be processed by computer systems.

- *Image pre-processing :*

Its aim is to improve these images when they contain noise or defects.

- *Image segmentation :*

Its aim is to build a symbolic image by generating homogeneous regions according to a criterion defined in advance.

- **Image analysis:** involves extracting parameters or functions representative of the image or regions.

These steps can be illustrated by a simple example [14].

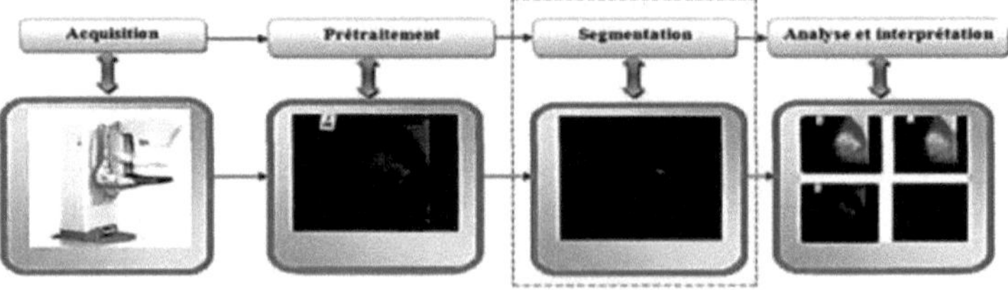

Figure 2.1: Steps in image processing.

2.1 Image pre-processing

A first step, often used, is to prepare the images before detection. As the structures we are looking for are not always easily discernible, a pre-processing step designed to highlight them can facilitate their detection [14].

Breast cancer (like all cancers in general) must be detected in its early phase to maximise the chances of survival. However, in this phase, it is very difficult to detect the pathology in the surrounding breast tissue with the naked eye without specific pre-processing of the image acquired. The main aim of this stage is therefore to increase the contrast between the breast lesion (whether a mass or microcalcifications) and the rest of the image to facilitate subsequent treatment. If a region of interest differs in luminance by less than 2% from the rest of the image, it remains indistinguishable from the naked eye (Dengler et al. 1993). The pre-processing of mammography images is known as enhancement or contrast enhancement.

2.2 Modification of mammogram histograms

a) Dynamic expansion :

modifying the histogram consists of distributing the pixel appearance frequencies over the width of the histogram to vary the contrasts in defined and different ways depending on the interval of (NG) considered. This transformation only improves the visual quality of the image, as the information present does not change.

b) Histogram equalisation

Histogram legalisation is a tool that is often useful for improving certain poor quality images (poor contrast, images that are too dark or too light, poor distribution of intensity levels, etc.) [15].

This transformation consists of making the histogram of the image's grey levels as flat as possible. We want each grey level to be equally represented in the image.

c) Histogram inversion :

This involves inverting the pixel values in relation to the average of the possible values. In a pathological mammography image, this operation allows opacities to be better visualised (black on a light background will be better perceived than white on a black background).

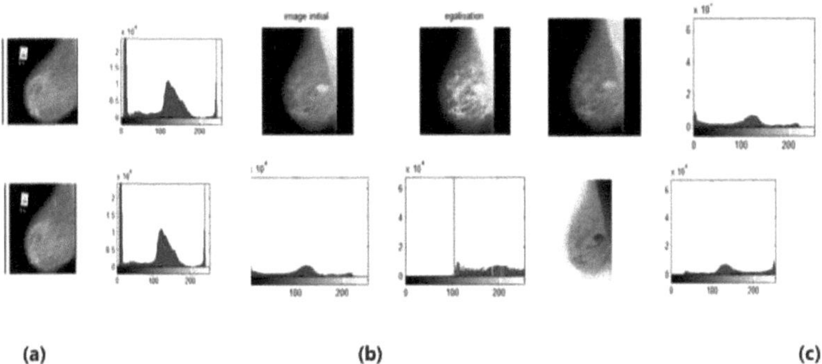

(a)   (b)   (c)

Figure2.2 Contrast enhancement techniques: (a) dynamic range expansion, (b) histogram equalization, (c) histogram inversion.

histogram equalisation, (c) histogram inversion.

2.3 Filtering mammograms

To improve the visual quality of an image, we need to eliminate the effects of noise by subjecting it to a process called filtering. Filtering is an operation that consists of applying a transformation to all or part of a digital image. The principle of filtering is to modify the value of pixels in an image, generally with the aim of improving its appearance [16].

2.3.1 Linear spatial filtering

a) *Low-pass filter (smoothing)*

This filter does not affect the low-frequency components in the image data, but should attenuate the high-frequency components.

b) *High-pass filter (emphasis)*

Contours are recessed and extracted in the frequency domain by applying a high-pass filter. The high-pass digital filter has the following characteristics

Inverse characteristics of the low-pass filter: It does not affect the high-frequency components of a signal, but must attenuate the low-frequency components.

c) *Gauss filter*

This is a low-pass linear filter. The values of the coefficients are determined according to a Gaussian function. The advantage of the Gaussian filter is that the degree of filtering can be easily adjusted via the standard deviation parameter.

Let A[x, y] be an original image and B[x, y] the filtered image such that :

B(x, y)=G(x, y)*A(x, y) **(2.1)**

2.3.2 Non-linear spatial filtering

a*) Median filter*

Averaging filters often tend to blur the image and therefore lose information on contours characterised by strong variations in intensity. To reduce this effect, we no longer average over the neighbourhood but take the median value over this neighbourhood: this is known as a median filter.

2.3.3 Morphological filtering

A morphological filter is an increasing and idempotent Φ operator:

x≤ *y*→Φ(*x*) ≤ Φ(y) Φ (Φ(*x*)) = Φ(*x*) **(2.2)**

Although the operations of dilation and erosion are not reversible, their succession makes it possible to develop two new morphological operations, namely opening and closing. [17]

a) *Morphological openness*

Of a set X, denoted XoB, is erosion by Bs followed by dilation with B :

X ° B= DBs (EB (X)) **(2.3)**

In any case, as we are using symmetrical elements, this amounts to performing the two operations with the same kernel. The opening is therefore :

X° B=DB (EB (X)) **(2.4)**

b) *Morphological closure*

Of a set X, denoted X·B, is the sequence of a dilation followed by an erosion by the same structuring element B :

X" B= EB (DB (X)) (2.5)

c) *Top hat transformation:*

The notion of top hat, due to F. Meyer, is a residue designed to eliminate slow variations in the signal, or to amplify contrasts. It therefore essentially applies to functions (digital images).

> White top hat (*WTH),*

Is defined as the algebraic difference between the identity (f) and its opening OB(f) such that:

WTHB(f)=f - OB(f) **(2.6)**

By symmetry, to extract the Vallès or highlight the dark structures in the image, we define

> *The black top hat:*

Black top hat (BTH) is defined as the algebraic difference between the closure FB(f) and the identity (f) such that :

BTHB(f)= FB(f) -f **(2.7)**

Figure (2.3) shows that the application of a white top hat makes it possible to
Detect all clear structures in the image (Mcs) :

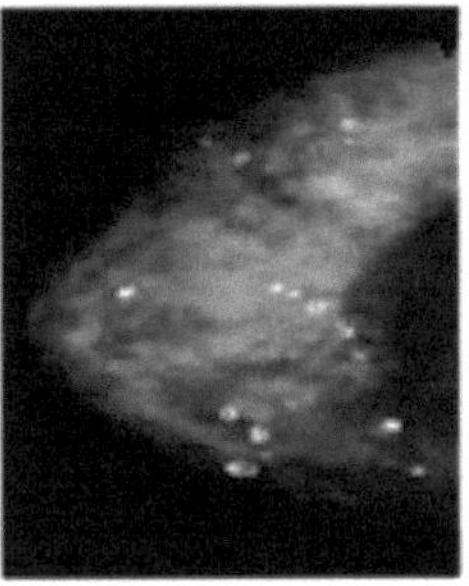
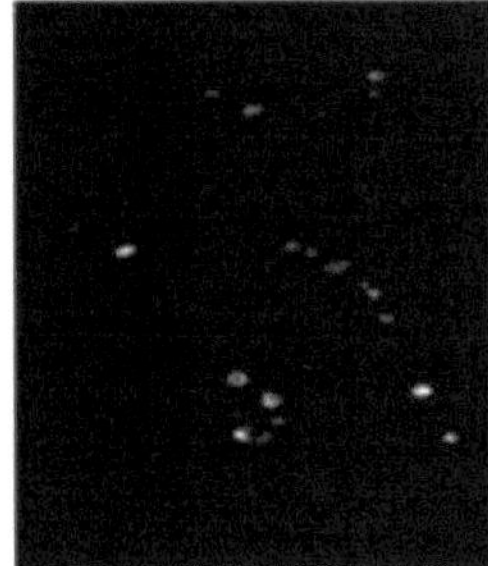

Figure2.3 Application of the "white top hat" transformation to NG mammography images
for the detection of breast lesions

d) *Sequential Alternate Filters :*

We define *Black Sequential Alternate Filter* of size n, denoted FASN(n), as an iteration of
successive openings and closings of increasing size. Such a filter is expressed as: *FASN (n)
=FnOn...F2O2 F1O1 (2.8)*

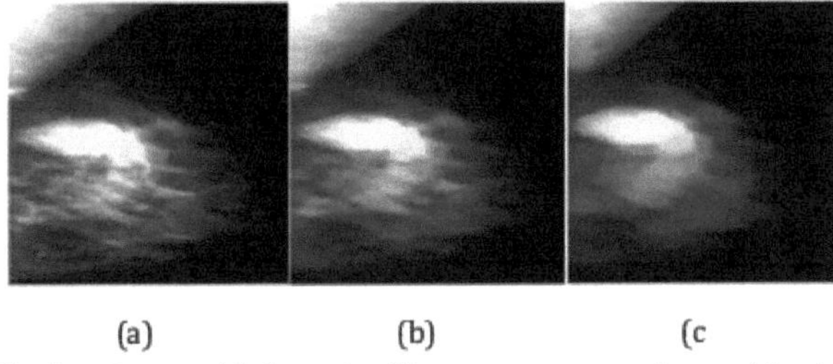

Figure 2.4 Application of sequential alternating filters to mammogram images (a) using size 2 (b) and
size 7 (c) structuring elements Mammogram segmentation

The aim of image analysis is to extract information such as shape, colour, contour, texture,
etc., and to do this, segmentation is one of the fundamental processes in the image processing
chain. Several techniques are proposed in the literature, each with its advantages and
disadvantages. We present 3 of the most widely used techniques applied to mammography:

- Contour-based segmentation approach.
- Regional segmentation approach.
- Segmentation by LPE.
- 4 Segmentation by classification.

3   *Purpose of segmentation*

The aim of image segmentation is to partition the image into areas of interest corresponding
to objectives in the scene from which it is taken. This provides a representation of the
information contained in the image and is a first step towards its interpretation. In the case of
medical image segmentation, the objective is **[18]** :

- Study anatomical structures.

- Identify regions of interest, tumour location, lesions and other abnormalities.
- Measurement of tissue volume to measure tumour growth.
- Helps plan treatment prior to radiology, by calculating the radiation dose.

The segmentation is based on [19] :

- A set of entities,
- a set of attributes characterising these entities,
- topological relationships between these entities,
- relational attributes.

We are looking for data partitions with intrinsic properties in relation to attributes and topological relationships (4-connectedness and 8-connectedness).

An image segmentation problem can therefore be characterised by a set of homogeneity criteria determining the properties of the image partitions we are looking for.

The criterion that defines homogeneity is therefore a determining factor in segmentation performance. The main criteria used are greyscale, colour for colour images and texture [19].

Numerous segmentation techniques have been proposed in the literature [19], but most of them require several parameters, the adjustment of which often requires human expertise.

4   The different segmentation approaches

There are many segmentation methods. In this section, we will present the various known techniques, organising them according to the approach that governs them. We have selected five approaches.

This classification and its further ramifications are shown in the figure below [20].

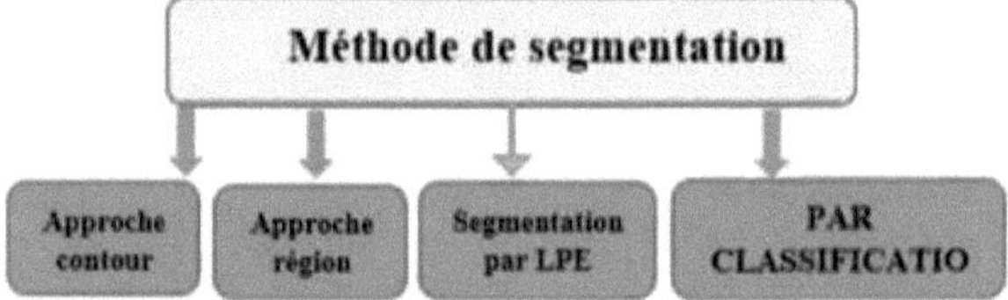

Figure 2.6. Classification of different segmentation methods

5.1 Segmentation by regional approach

Region-based segmentation is an approach in which surfaces are constructed by grouping neighbouring pixels according to a homogeneity criterion [21].

Segmentation by region creates a set of regions with the following properties:

- Putting all the regions together gives the whole image.
- Regions are related, i.e. all pixels in the same region are contiguous.
- All the pixels in the same region are homogeneous.

This approach differs, for example, from edge-based or threshold-based segmentations in which the regions created do not all have these properties. The following methods can be distinguished within this approach:

Adjacent similar regions are merged with the starting seeds, resulting in larger regions. Considering the regions thus obtained, the process is then iterated until the number of regions likely to be merged is exhausted [22].

A set of regions with the following properties:

- Putting all the regions together gives the whole image.
- Regions are related, i.e. all pixels in the same region are contiguous.

·   All the pixels in the same region are homogeneous.

This approach distinguishes between the following methods:

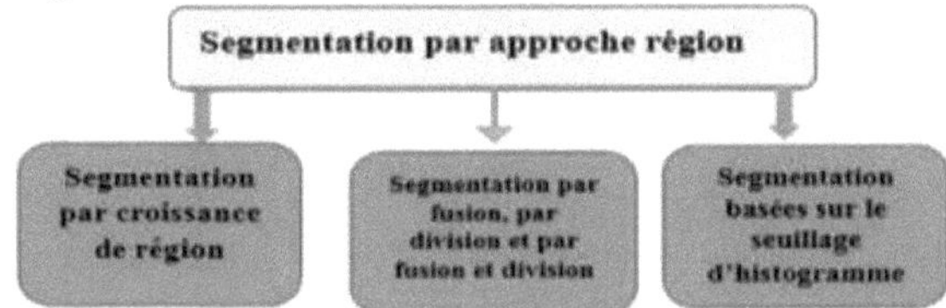

Figure 2.7. Different segmentation methods using a regional approach

5.1.1 Region growth methods

Region-growth segmentation methods are based on the use of seed points, which are chosen either manually or automatically. These seeds designate the starting points or regions within the image to be segmented. Using similarity measures, each seed is compared with its immediate spatial neighbourhood. Based on these similarity measures, adjacent similar regions are merged with the starting seeds, resulting in larger regions. Considering the regions thus obtained, the process is then iterated until all the regions likely to be merged are exhausted **[22]**.

* ***The algorithm is globally :***
* choice of regional seeds.
* gradual integration of neighbouring pixels into each sprout.
* a pixel is conquered if the difference between its NG and the average NG for the region is faible

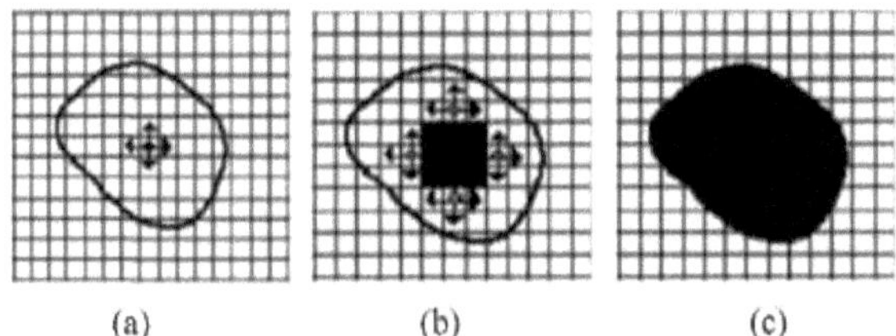

(a)   (b)   (c)

Figure 2.8 The process of a region growth algorithm. (a)Sprout. (b) Aggregation process after a few iterations. (c) The segmentation result.

5.1.2 Approach based on merging and dividing regions

a- Split segmentation :

These approaches divide the original image into smaller regions according to a heterogeneity criterion. Cutting stops when there are no more inhomogeneous regions **[23]**.

The principle of this technique is to consider the image itself as the initial region, which is then divided into regions. The division process is repeated for each new region (resulting from the division) until homogeneous classes are obtained **[24]**.

b- Segmentation by merging regions (Merge)

Region merging techniques are bottom-up methods in which all pixels are visited.

These methods operate by grouping pixels or groups of pixels according to a homogeneity criterion to obtain a set of homogeneous regions **[25]**. They follow a tree-like hierarchy.

Several grouping rules have been proposed in the literature. Some of these rules involve :

Statistical properties such as the mean or variance of the grey levels of the regions, the mean gradient of the borders of the regions, the maximum contrast of the regions, or other local statistics that express the state of the surface of the regions;

• Geometric or morphological properties such as the elongation or compactness of regions. Two regions are grouped together if, for example, a form factor is retained or improved after they are merged.

c- Split and Merge segmentation

Proposed by Horowitz [26], they bring together all the algorithms used in the above techniques (fusion methods and division methods).

The segmentation process takes place in two stages:

• Iteratively divide the image by exploiting the specific characteristics of each region according to a heterogeneity criterion (surface, light intensity, colourimetry, texture, etc.) until we have blocks containing exclusively similar pixels.

• Merge neighbouring blocks if they are similar and repeat the operation until the characteristics of the image meet a predefined condition: number of regions, brightness, contrast or texture.

5.1.3 Segmentation methods based on histogram thresholding

These are basic image segmentation methods [27]. The general principle of thresholding is to look for an appropriate threshold value and then classify all the pixels in the image according to the value of their grey levels in relation to this threshold in order to separate the regions of interest and the image background.

Generally speaking, thresholding methods can be classified into two categories:

a- Global thresholding methods

It is considered to be the reference method in the field of histogram thresholding. These methods are widely used in mammography image segmentation to detect tumour areas or calcifications. [28].

The principle of this method is to separate the pixels of an image into two classes !

(background), " (object) based on a threshold S. The "background" class contains all pixels with a grey level below the threshold S, while the "object" class contains all pixels with a grey level above S. [29].

b- Local thresholding methods

These methods aim to refine the threshold value locally to better identify the regions of interest. The threshold value is determined by limiting the information contained in the local neighbourhood of each pixel [30]. These methods have often shown better detection efficiency than global thresholding methods. Note that local thresholding methods have not only been used for image segmentation, but have also been exploited as a dedicated pre-processing step for other algorithms such as those based on Markov fields [30].

5.2 Contour segmentation :

A contour is a set of pixels forming a boundary between two or more neighbouring regions. The thickness of a contour is one or more pixels and it is defined by a "rapid" variation in characteristics.

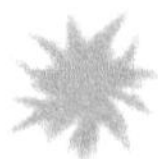

(a)- Edges   (b)- Edges (c)- Edges   (d)- Edges   (e)- Speculated edges
Circumscribed erased micro-lobulated ill-defined

Figure 2.9: Schematic representation of mass contours

In general, a regular, round, oval or lobulated opacity that is well limited and has a clear contour is not cause for concern, as these are a priori benign lesions. However, this rule is not absolute, as some cancers can have the same characteristics. However, an abnormal opacity with a hyperdense centre; unclear and irregular boundaries are signs of suspected malignancy. [31]

Edge extraction methods are based on the detection of discontinuities in the image and can be divided into three classes:

* derivative methods ;
* analytical methods ;
* methods based on active contours.

We can cite approaches based on the derivative method, such as the gradient operation,

The Laplacian operation and various filters such as the sobel, prewitt and roberts filters or analytical approaches such as the canny filter. These types of techniques are not very useful because they can give unclosed contours and remain sensitive to noise. The third approach for detecting contours is proposed by active contours (snakes). This method will be described in detail later. [**31**].

5.2.1 Deformable models

In recent years, deformable models, one of the most popular contour segmentation methods, have been widely used in image segmentation. The idea behind deformable models is quite simple. The user determines an initial estimate for the contour which is then deformed by forces derived from the image until the desired objects are delineated.

Two main types of deformable models can be distinguished: [**32**]

* **Parametric deformable models**
* **Geometric deformable models**

5.2.2 6.2.2 Parametric deformable models

a- Active contour (snake)

Active snake contours are closed curves laid out on an image that we want to converge on a particular area of the image by moving them iteratively. These curves are defined in the image domain, and can move under the influence of forces internal to the curve and external forces calculated from the image data. An internal energy (E Int) which depends solely on the shape of the snake and represents a constraint on the regularity of the curve. A potential energy (E image) linked to the image, characterising the elements of the image (I) to which the snake must be attracted. A constraint energy (Econt) linked to the problem; for example, the minimum distance between two points on the snake or the snake's passage through control points. [33]

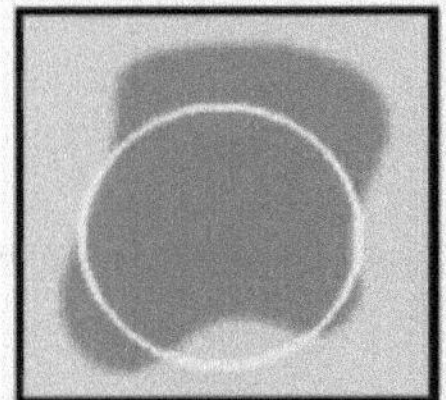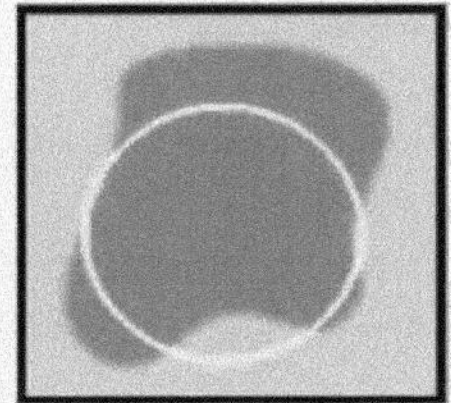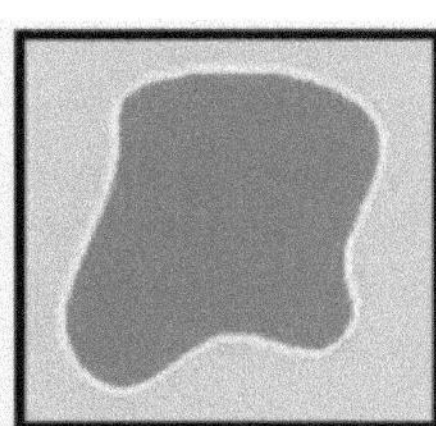

Figure 2.10: Active contour principle

5.2.3 Geometric deformable models

a- Level set segmentation

The method of Zero Level Sets is a numerical simulation method used for the evolution of curves and surfaces in discrete domains.

The basic idea behind the levelset method is to consider a curve (or interface) in motion as the zero level of a higher-dimensional function. For a 2D Curve, this interface (Ψ) is the intersection of a hyper surface (of dimension 3) with A plane

The points defining this interface will move towards the normal at a speed F according to the following equation **[34]** :

$$Tt+1+F[_{ATt}]=0 \quad (2.9)$$

This velocity F is composed of three terms: a constant term (similar to the inflation force used in deformable models), a term depending on the local curvature

At each point and an image-dependent term (in our case, the image edges).

The numerical diagram of the interface displacement equation is described by equation :

$$T_{n+1}=T_n - dt*k_1(x,y)*(U_n - s\ K)*[AT_l]\ s \in [0, 1] \quad (2.10)$$

With :

$Un(m, \sigma) = \pm 1$, membership function defining the zone or object to be searched.

$K = A.[AT/AT]$, local curvature at each point of the interface

$kI(x,y)$, a stopping criterion dependent on the gradient image.

Initialization is performed with one or more starting shapes.

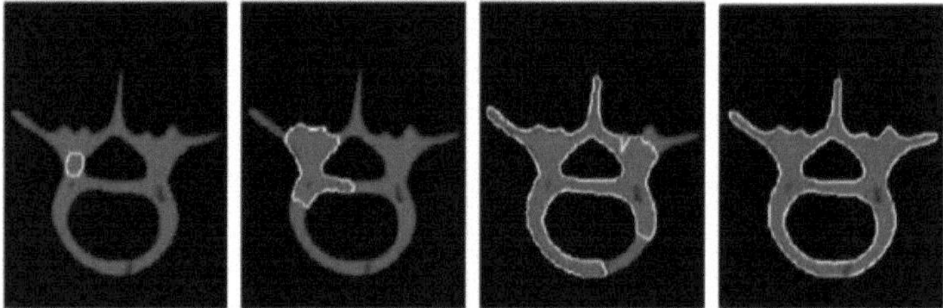

Figure 2.11: Level Sets principle

The main advantage of this method is the ability to automatically manage the change in topology of the evolving curve.

And its limitations:

- Divergence problem: Resolution method.
- Interpolation: loss of material.
- Calculation cost: Resetting the distance function.

5.3 Segmentation by watershed (LPE)

The Watershed (LPE) uses a description of images in geographical terms (Fig. 2.12). It does not apply to the original image, but to the image of its

Morphological gradient where the grey level of each point corresponds to an altitude. It is then possible to define the watershed as the ridge forming the boundary between two catchment areas. A catchment area is a geographical zone from which a drop of water, following the line of greatest slope, will arrive at a given minimum. A minimum is associated with a catchment area. [35]

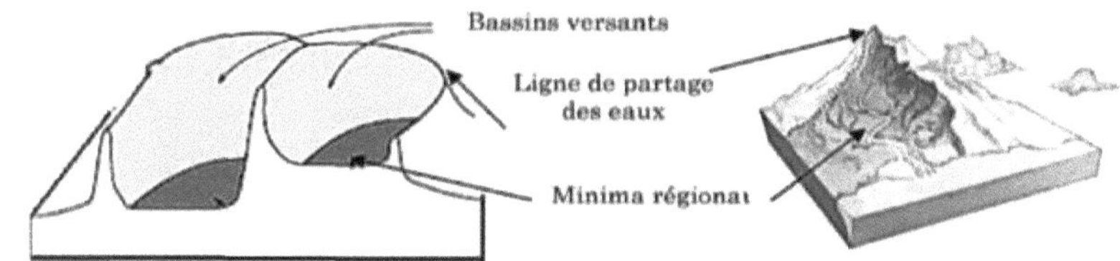

Figure2.12 Tomographic characteristics of a digital image

Generally, to describe this algorithm, the flooding processes, a particular description of the image seen as a topographic relief :
We can imagine that this topographic surface is perforated at the locations of the minima (Fig. 2.13). Let's slowly immerse this surface in a lake (watershed). The water will flow through the holes (i.e. the local minima). So that the water level rises at a constant speed and is uniform throughout the catchment area.
When the waters from two different minima meet, a dam is built to prevent them from mixing.
When the entire topographic surface has been swallowed up, only the dams will emerge, delimiting the catchment areas as local minima of the f function.
These dams form the watershed.

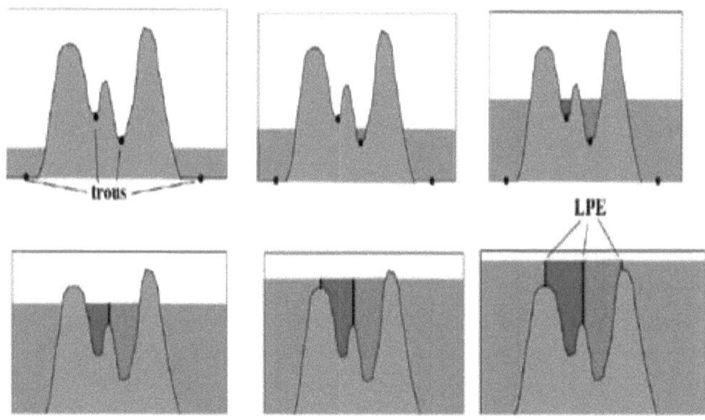

Figure2.13 The EPL construction process

However, applying the LPE algorithm to natural images produces over-segmentation. To avoid this phenomenon, the EPL topology must be constrained.

5.3.1 The EPL Under the constraint of markers

The principle of the homotopy modification of the gradient is to impose the markers of the Regions to be segmented as minima of the gradient by deleting all the other undesirable minima which are at the origin of any over-segmentation (Fig. 2.14). This Gradient is then flooded with all the markers. One and only one dividing line is then present between each marker, and it tends to lie on the contour of the objects to be segmented, which have already been pre-detected by the gradient.

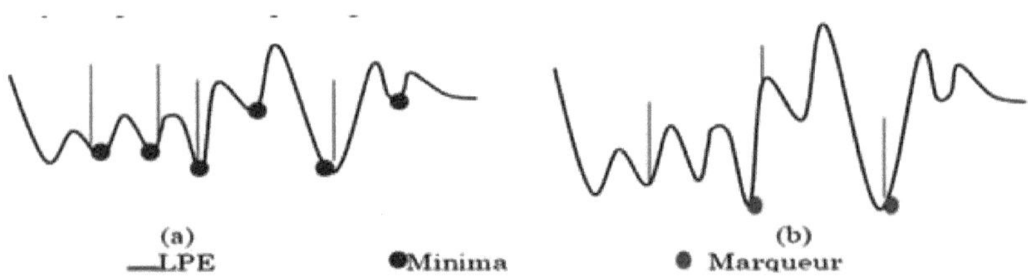

Figure 2.14 Flooding LPE process with stress (b) and without stress (a)

5.4 Segmentation by classification :

Among image segmentation techniques, classification is one of the most widely used procedures. Image classification consists of partitioning the image into a set of a disjoint classes. There are two approaches to image classification: _ The supervised approach. The unsupervised approach

6   Superficial overview of some works for the detection of breast lesions :

In diagnostic aid systems (DAS), the segmentation of breast masses and microcalcifications is an important and delicate task, given that the subsequent description, classification and registration processes are strictly linked to the segmentation result. Consequently, good detection of the lesion contour produces a description that is faithful to its characteristics. As a result, we can ensure a classification that minimises the rate of false positives and maximises the rate of true negatives.

However, it has been shown that the detection of masses is more difficult than the detection of SAMs (Malagelada, 2007). Indeed, it is difficult to distinguish masses from normal regions due to their low contrast and ambiguous edges partially masked by tissue. [35]

Thresholding methods have made a considerable contribution to the segmentation of

Breast masses (Kom et al. 2007; Kurt et al. 2014).

(Mudigonda et al., 2001) used multi-level thresholding to detect closed contours. The major drawback of this approach is that it assumes that the masses have a uniform density relative to the image background, which is not always verified (Cheikhrouhou, 2012).

Another work in the same context is (Kai et al. 2017) where the authors performed a two-stage adaptive thresholding (DuSAT). A global thresholding which focuses on the analysis of the histogram peaks (HPA) of the whole image, the threshold is obtained by maximising the proposed thresholding criterion. Local thresholding is then performed for each pixel in a defined neighbourhood window to provide accurate segmentation results [35].

Very recently, Anitha and her team (Anitha et al. 2017) proceeded in the same way as Kai (Kai et al. 2011). Other methods have been proposed and were based on wavelet transforms to improve the contrast of mammography images (Vikhe and Thoul, 2016) before the application of an adaptive thresholding technique. To extract the tumour region the authors in (Elmoufidi et al. 2017) used local binary patterns (LBP) which compare the luminance level of a pixel with the levels of its neighbours.

This therefore provides texture information [35].

Morphological segmentation using watershed lines has attracted a great deal of interest in the image processing community and numerous studies have proven the effectiveness of this method in detecting breast masses (Hsu, 2012).

As discussed earlier, EPL first involves a pre-processing step to avoid over-segmentation. As a result, after a morphological filtering step (Anuradha et al. 2015) proposed classical EPL applied on the gradient of the filtered image to obtain mass contours.

(Dubey et al. 2010) have demonstrated the effectiveness of EPL for mass detection in terms of speed and accuracy by comparing it with a semi-automatic approach based on sets of levels [35].

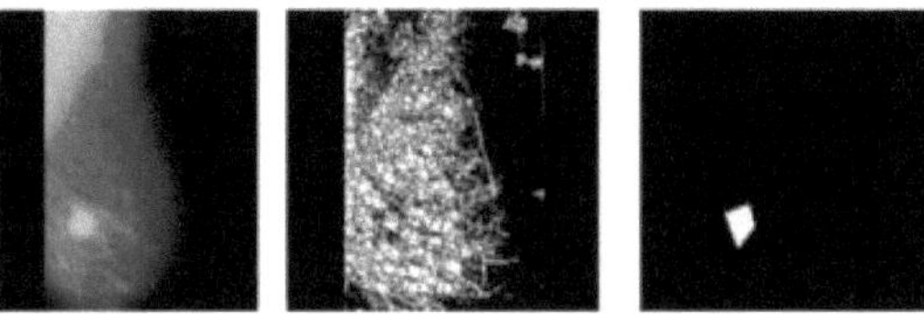

FIGURE 2.15 Segmentation steps proposed by (Anuradha et al, 2015): from left to right, initial image, Watershed gradient and markers, breast mass detection.

The region growth technique has been used by various researchers (Berber et al. ,2012; Melouah, 2015), all of whom note that preprocessing is necessary For good contour convergence (Figure 2.15).

The authors in (Görgel et al. 2013) first used homomorphic filtering in their approach to improve image contrast and then the region growth method to find mass-like tumour regions.

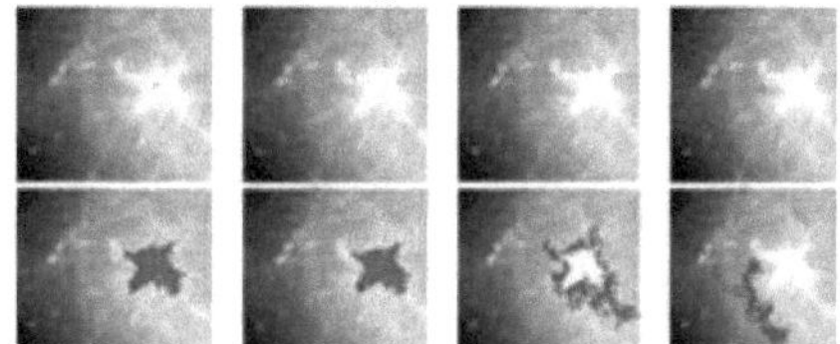

FIGURE 2.16 Examples of different germ positions of the approach proposed by (Melouah, 2015) and the result obtained.

In the case of contour approaches, the researchers in (Lu et al. 2015) used active contours for mass detection. First, they performed a pre-processing step to remove film artefacts and improve image contrast. They then

Using the circular Hough transform to detect the mass contour. This is used as the initial contour to start the active contours process.

An alternative to region-growth methods is segmentation by splitting and merging. This approach has not been sufficiently exploited in the context of breast mass segmentation.

A new technique for segmenting fibro-glandular tissue has been proposed by (Reyad et al. 2013), based on the "divide and merge" technique applied to the histogram of the mammographic image. The main difficulty of this approach lies in traversing the set of all pairs of neighbouring regions and setting the stopping criterion for the method (Cheikhrouhou, 2012). [35]

7 *Conclusion*

In this chapter, we have proposed a classification of methods for segmenting mammography images, explaining the best-known and most widely used techniques. However, each of them has its qualities, and it is on this basis that the choice of using one or other of these techniques should be made...?

An analysis of the principles and performance of the various segmentation methods leads to the following conclusions:

- Region-growth segmentation methods based on grey-level measurements (including textural measurements) or probabilistic measurements provide good initial identification of the regions of interest, but suffer from the major disadvantage of imprecise location of the contours of these regions.
- The active contour segmentation approach gives good results in terms of locating the contours of the regions of interest, provided that the initialization of these contours is not too far from the final contours. However, the textured nature of mammography images often results in multiple false contours within the detected regions.
- Segmentation methods based on the watershed concept are powerful and flexible, but the choice of parameters remains the weak link in this method.

Chapter 3

RESULTS AND INTERPRETATION

1 Introduction

Mammography images play a vital role in the detection of breast tumours, providing radiological information such as the nature, type and condition of the tumour, and if we can detect all this information we can improve the patient's vital prognosis.

Researchers are keen to develop computer diagnosis/detection systems to detect this type of cancer in its early stages, in order to maximise the chances of survival.

At this stage, however, it is very difficult to identify the pathology in the surrounding breast tissue with the naked eye without specific pre-processing of the image acquired.

Why do we detect breast opacities?

- quantitative parameters to determine the nature of the lesions: According to the standard

- Breast opacities must be detected in their early phase to maximise the chances of survival.

- Reduce the error made by radiologists: The classification of breast lesions by a radiologist is a subjective human classification that can easily classify the same lesion in two different ways.

- Help radiologists with their interpretations: Several studies have shown that radiologists miss between 4% and 38% of cancer detections, and that this rate improves by 15% by using a second reading, given that interpretation is often difficult and depends on the radiologist's expertise.

As a result, in this chapter we mainly propose the different methods of image processing based on mathematical morphology and segmentation approaches to ensure better quality in terms of the needs and performance of the subsequent algorithms.

2 Database

In this work, we use the mini-Mias (Mammography Image Analysis Society) image database [36]. MIAS is an organisation of mammography research groups in the United Kingdom which has developed a database of digital mammograms with a spatial resolution of 1024*1024 pixels for each image. This database contains 322 images divided into 207 normal images, 38 images containing masses and 169 containing other abnormalities.

3 Pre-treatment

The idea of pre-processing, although intuitive, can solve the problems of mammography artefacts. It is a step designed to highlight them, which can facilitate their detection and improve image quality. Ideally, we would like to highlight only the potentially suspicious areas in order to facilitate their detection at a later date. However, in order to carry out this task, we need to know which areas of the image need to be enhanced, i.e. we need to know which areas are suspect, which is difficult because we are trying to enhance the image precisely to detect these structures. Similarly, pre-processing can substantially modify the properties of the image, making it difficult to model the detection stage.

The purpose of the pre-processing step is to facilitate segmentation by reinforcing the similarity between pixels belonging to the same region, or by accentuating the dissimilarity between pixels belonging to different regions.

3.1 Artefacts in mammography

This background may contain artefacts that the human visual system can easily ignore during interpretation, but an automated system must first identify and classify these artefacts, which cause interpretation errors during image analysis [37]. A number of

CAD systems currently work on digitised mammograms. Radioactive artefacts often appear on such images (fig3.1).

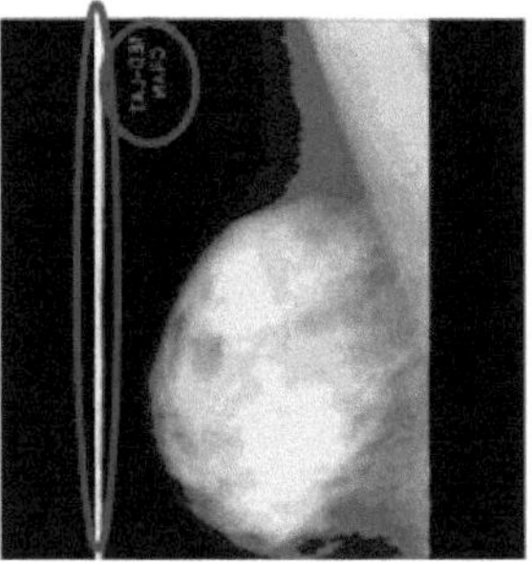 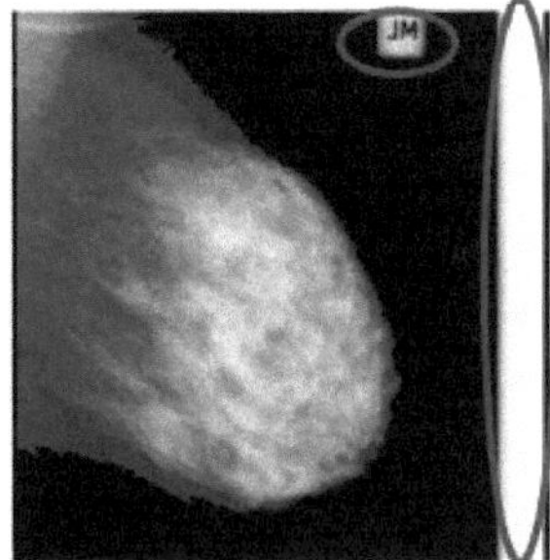

Figure3.1 artefacts in a mammography image

3.2 Mammography film labels

Mammograms are generally marked with some form of permanent identification label containing information about the examination performed [37]. These labels are radiopaque indicators showing the laterality of the mammogram.

(R/L, Right/Left) and MLO /CC1 projection indicators (Fig3.2).

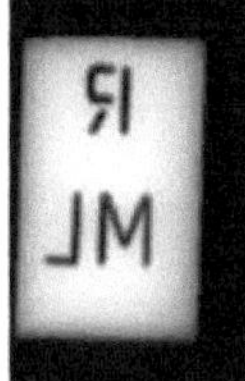 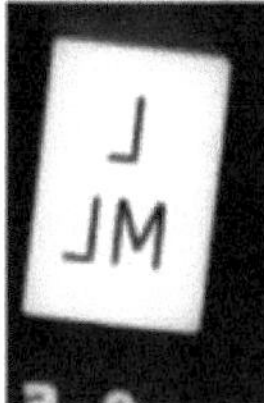

Figure3.2 Mammography film labels

3.3 Radiopaque artefacts

There are two types of radiopaque artefacts: high intensity bands or wedges and opaque markers (fig3.3). These markers are labels where the text is in high intensity (the rectangle surrounding the text does not exist). Corners are high-intensity bands that run along the edge of the mammogram [37].

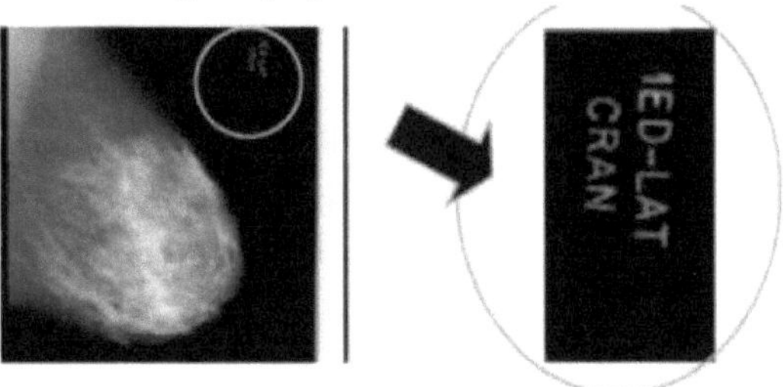

Figure3.3 Opaque markers

3.4 The reasons for digitisation

A line is a local extremum of high intensity (light or dark) parallel to the abscissa axes

(Fig3.4).

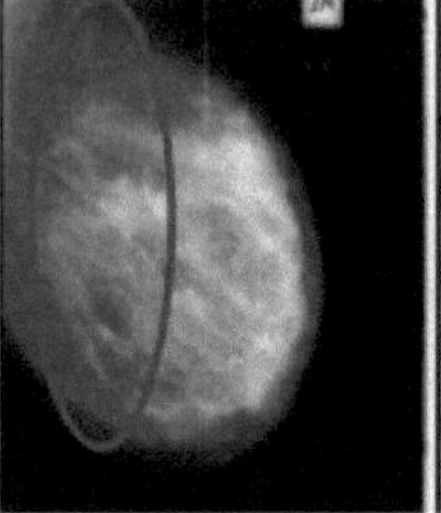

Figure3.4 scanning lines

4   *Proposed approach to mammary gland extraction*

The aim of our approach is to extract or isolate the 'breast' region of interest from the initial volume of data (the mammography image), while at the same time removing all types of noise.

The algorithm is based on the application of morphological filters to remove any noise.

Then, a carefully chosen threshold reveals two related regions of very different sizes. Surface filtering is used to create the mask corresponding to the mammary gland. From this mask and the filtered image, we recover the region of interest and the background of the cleaned mammogram.

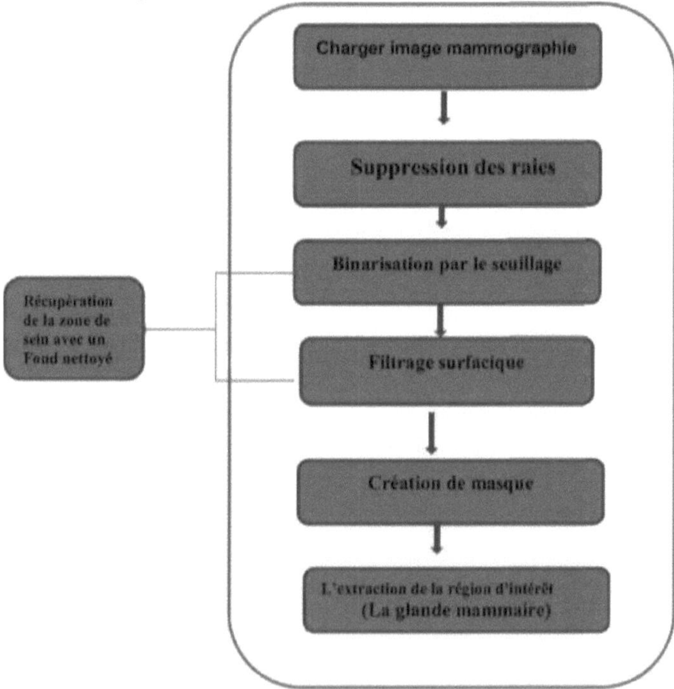

Figure 3.5 Pre-treatment stages

4.1 Removal of lines :

Removing scan lines from an image (Fig3.6.a) is complicated because they often cover the breast area.

We propose a simple method based on the application of two types of morphological filters: opening and closing. In our case, they are well suited since we know the shape and contrast of the structures to be removed.

> ^Removal of light line using morphological opening by Se=2
> Suppression of dark lines using morphological closure with Se=4

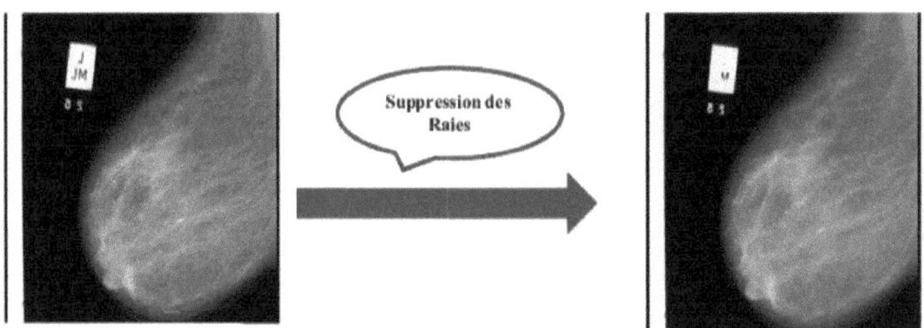

Figure 3.6: Scanning line suppression results for the mdb147 image

4.2 Recovery of the breast area with a cleaned bottom

Once the scan lines have been eliminated, the 2nd step consists of eliminating background artefacts (labels, radio opaque artefacts, high intensity bands on the edges). The steps in this 2nd part consist of three stages: thresholding to isolate objects from the background; surface filtering to obtain the mask and, finally, recovery of the area of interest.

4.2.1 Filtering the filtered image

After primary cleaning of the mammographic image, the mammary gland and other structures (radio-opaque artefacts, labels on the X-ray film, etc.) are extracted from the filtered image using a well-chosen threshold (Fig. 3.7).

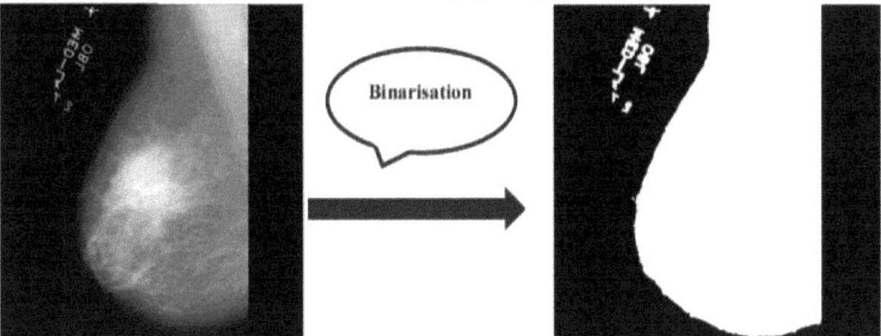

Figure 3.7: Thresholding result.

4.2.2 Creating the breast mask

After the binarisation step, several related objects are obtained, such as radiopaque artefacts, labels and the breast. A simple surface filtering is applied to create a mask of the region of interest, the breast (Fig3.8).

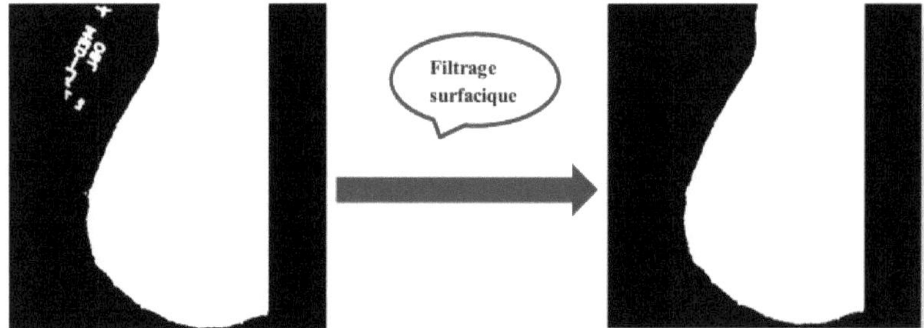

Figure 3.8: Surface filtering result

4.2.3 Extraction of the region of interest (the mammary gland)

To recover the region of interest, a simple arithmetic multiplication is calculated between the values of the previous mask pixels and the result of the filtering step. The contour obtained by our pre-segmentation method is superimposed on the filtered images.

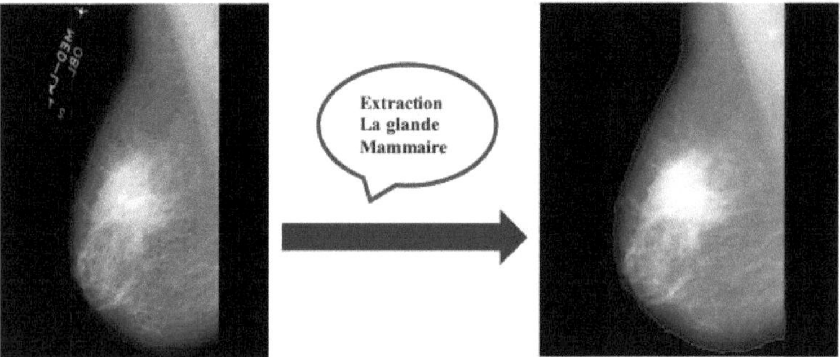

Figure 3.9 Final result of mammary gland extraction.

4.2.4 Results and discussion

In this pre-processing phase, our aim is to reduce execution time, and to make the segmentation tasks more efficient, we apply our pre-processing algorithm, which consists of extracting the "mammary gland" zone of interest.

We tested this pre-processing step on the MIAS database containing 322 mammograms: 110 images did not contain radio-opaque artefacts, but suffered from a noisy background, and 212 images contained the radio-opaque artefacts mentioned above in the form of identification labels, opaque markers and lines.

This algorithm is parametric, and is not sensitive to the size of the mammary gland, its density or the size of these artefacts, or to their positions and orientations. The knowledge required for initialisation is the average grey level on a digital mammogram, and the size of the scanning lines.

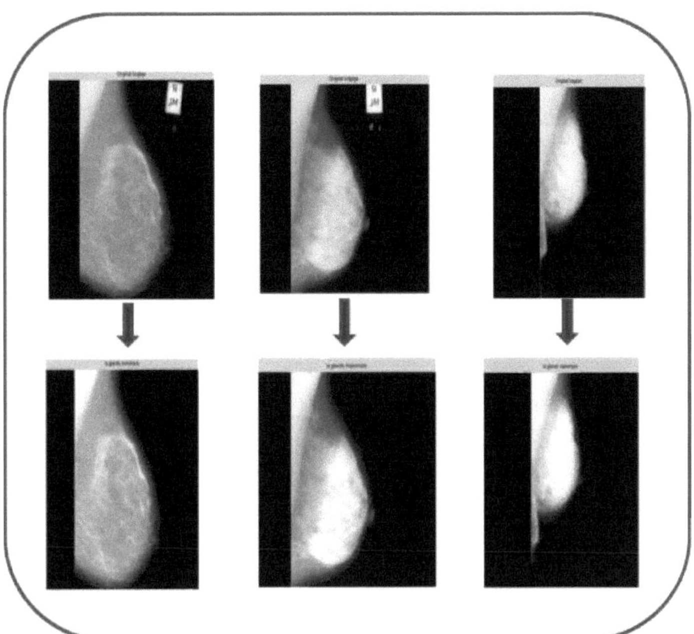

Figure 3.10: Extraction of the mammary gland from the various MIAS images

Visually, the results are acceptable, and when we apply these results to all the mammography images in the MIAS database, we can move on to the second part of this chapter, 'mass segmentation'.

5 Breast mass segmentation strategies

Detecting breast masses is an important task in the early diagnosis of breast cancer. This difficulty is largely due to the complexity of mammographic images (breast density) and the diversity of opacities to be segmented. Taking these difficulties into account.

The main stages of mass detection proposed in this chapter are illustrated in the following figure:

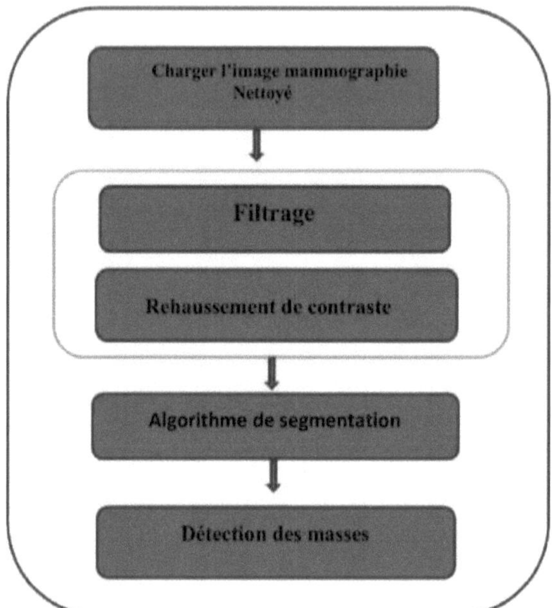

Figure 3.11: The main steps in breast mass detection algorithms.

The input mammography image is a cleaned image using the technique proposed in the first part (Mammography image pre-processing). After loading, the image undergoes pre-processing (a filtering step and a contrast enhancement step) to reduce noise and improve contrast. Segmentation algorithms are then applied to detect masses. The various stages of the algorithm are then described in detail.

5.1 Filtering :

To improve the visual quality of mammographic images, because the images they represent are altered in relation to the scenes they represent, with noise of various origins being added to them. The same scene will therefore appear differently depending on the type of sensor used, the spatial resolution or the spectral band considered.

This noise is generally the cause of errors in detecting objects in images. Because of this, we have to eliminate the effects of the noise (parasites) by subjecting it to a process called filtering.

5.1.1 The different types of filter

✓ *Linear filtering :*

Linear filters use a window (mask) containing coefficients. Filtering is performed by convolving the image with this mask. The result is a smoothed image, which can be useful for reducing the noise present in the image, but the disadvantage is that it performs this smoothing on the entire image; the contours will therefore be smoothed, becoming blurred, although the interior of objects is not desirable [38].

✓ *Low-pass filter*: reduces noise but attenuates image detail.

✓ *High-pass filter:* accentuates the contours and details of the image but increases noise.

✓ **_Band-pass filter_**: Eliminates certain undesirable frequencies present in the image

✓ **_Gauss filter_**

This is a low-pass linear filter. The values of the coefficients are determined according to a Gaussian function. The advantage of the Gaussian filter is that the degree of filtering can be easily adjusted via the standard deviation parameter.

Let A[x, y] be an original image and B[x, y] the filtered image such that :

B(x, y)=G(x, y)*A(x, y) **(3.1)**

✓ **_Non-linear spatial filtering_**

✓ **_Median filter_**

Averaging filters often tend to blur the image and therefore lose information on contours characterised by strong variations in intensity. To reduce this effect, we no longer average over the neighbourhood but take the median value over this neighbourhood: this is known as a median filter.

✓ **_Morphological filtering_**

✓ **_Sequential Alternate Filters :_**

We define _Black Sequential Alternate Filter_ of size n, denoted FASN(n), as an iteration of successive openings and closings of increasing size. Such a filter is expressed as :

FASN (n) =FnOn...F2O2 F1O1 **(3.2)**

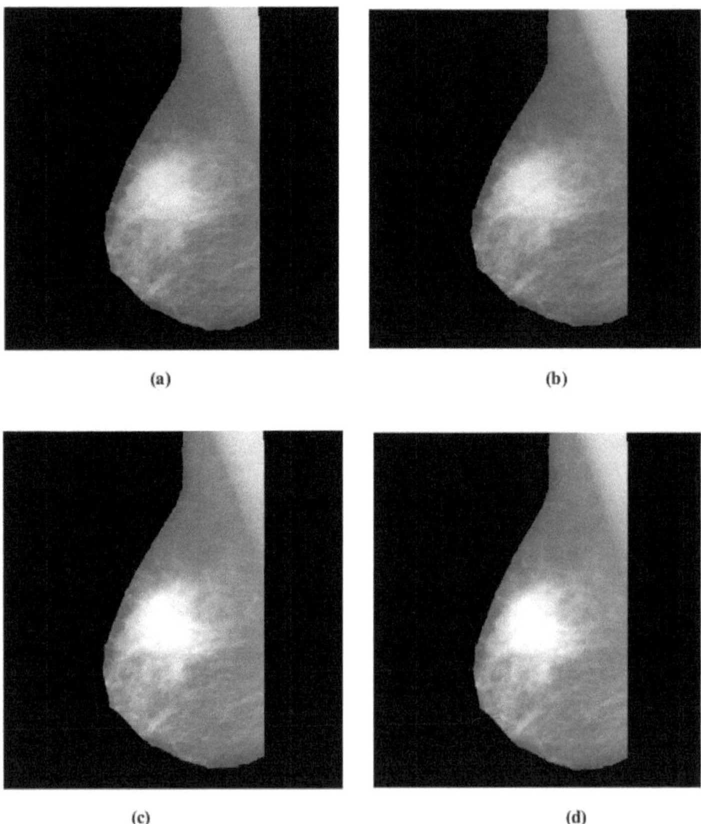

(a)   (b)

(c)   (d)

FIGURE 3.12 Performance of different proposed filtering approaches on pathological mammography images: (a) Original image, (b) Median filter (c) Gaussian filter (e) Sequential Alternate filter

5.1.2 Objective assessment of the quality of the filters developed

Among the range of measures used in the literature, the quantitative measures commonly used are the mean square error (MSE) and the peak signal to noise ratio (PSNR). These two criteria are used to quantify the quality of denoising and to test the effectiveness of each filter on mammographic images in order to arrive at a correct choice of the most suitable filter for our images.

- Root mean square error: (RMSE) is calculated between the pixels of the original image I and the pixels of the degraded image[14] of size m x n, in order to determine the similarity ratio:

$$EQM = \frac{1}{M \times N} \sum_{m=1}^{M} \sum_{n=1}^{N} (I(m,n) - \hat{I}(m,n))^2 \qquad (3.3)$$

The peak signal-to-noise ratio (PSNR) is determined from this value:

40

$$PSNR = 10\log_{10}\left(\frac{I^2_{max}}{EQM}\right) \qquad (3.4)$$

Or: Imax is the maximum possible luminance

However, it is known in the image processing literature that a processed image of good quality (compared to the original image) has typical PSNR values varying between 30 dB and 40 dB (Gomes, 2008).

In our case, these two criteria were evaluated for the three proposed filtering approaches and the results obtained are presented in the following table:

Filtering	Median filter	Gaussian filter	Alternate filters
EQM	0.1284 E -04	6.9829e+03	3,81E-04
PSNR	57.0440	9.6904	34,6

Table 1. Comparison of EQM and PSNR values for the different filters

In view of these results, the median filter provides a good compromise between noise reduction (PSNR) and edge preservation (EQM). In a dense mammographic image, the median filter is the best suited, offering an excellent PSNR= **57.0440** (dB) ratio (very little loss) and the lowest value for the parameter (MSE=0.**1284 E -04**).

The linear Gaussian filter offers relatively low PSNR values compared with the Alternate filter. As a result, the type of filtering best suited to our images for

denoising is the median filter. It is the one that provides a good compromise between noise reduction and the preservation of object contours.

5.2 Contrast enhancement

After filtering the image, a contrast enhancement is performed to highlight all the high-frequency spots, in other words all the regions likely to be masses.

The problem with contrast enhancement algorithms is that some regions may not be properly enhanced while others may be over-enhanced. A lack of contrast enhancement can cause false negatives. Many details of the lesion may be overlooked. In this case, certain lesions may go undetected and subsequently undiagnosed. This does not meet the main objective of early cancer detection. Excessive contrast enhancement can cause false positives. In this case, several details that do not really exist may be added to the lesion. As a result, certain normal areas of breast tissue may be considered as lesions, leading to unnecessary biopsies. The global histogram modification approach is used to improve these contrast problems. This method consists of reassigning the intensity values of the pixels in order to make the new intensity distribution more uniform. This can be achieved by histogram equalisation [39].

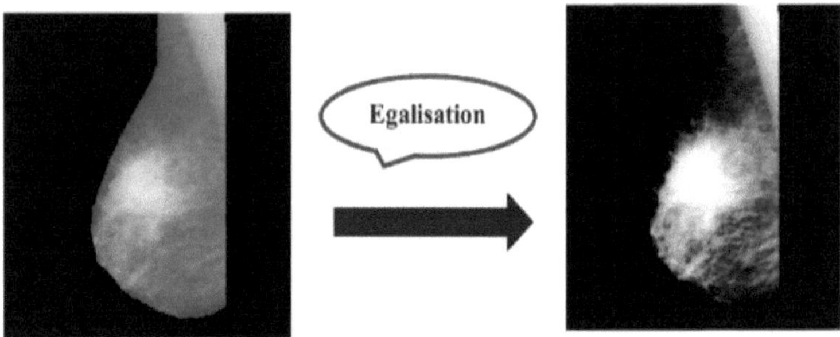

Figure 3.13: Histogram equalisation result

5.3 Image segmentation

Image segmentation can be considered as low-level processing; its aim is to extract elements from the image and consists of partitioning the image into homogeneous regions according to one or more criteria [40]. Each group of pixels then forms a region. A region is therefore a connected set of pixels with common properties (intensity, texture, etc.) that differentiate them from pixels in neighbouring regions. It is generally only an essential first step in the process of interpreting a scene.

5.3.1 Different approaches to mammography segmentation

Essentially, the aim of image analysis is to extract the characteristic information contained in an image. This information can take the form of shape, colour, contour, etc. It is therefore necessary first to segment the lesion by subdividing it into regions

There are a number of segmentation techniques available for this subdivision into distinct homogeneous regions. These methods are commonly classified into three categories: pixel-based approaches, contour-based approaches and region-based approaches. Pixel-based approaches are generally based on the study of image histograms using thresholding, clustering or fuzzy clustering. Contour-based approaches approach segmentation as a search for boundaries between objects (anomalies) and the background. They involve identifying pixel intensity transitions between regions to define the edges of the anomalies being sought. Region-based approaches involve partitioning the image into distinct regions of a certain homogeneity. Several techniques are proposed in the literature, each with its advantages and disadvantages. We present the three techniques most commonly used in mammography.

> **Segmentation by morphology (The Watershed).**
> **Segmentation by region (regional growth).**
> **Segmentation by classification (K-means). >**

5.3.2 Morphological segmentation (The watershed)

The main detection strategy proposed in this approach is illustrated in the following figure : Figure 3.17

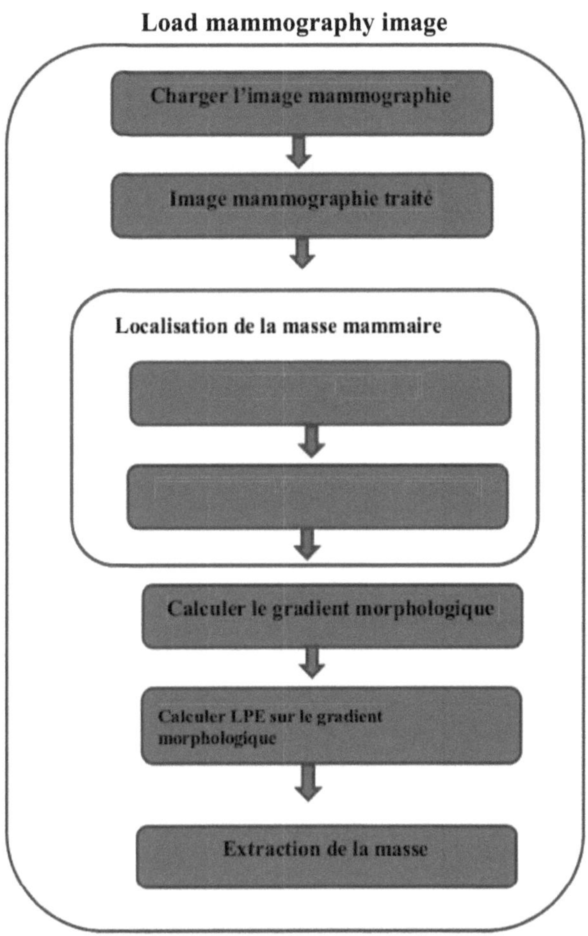

Figure 3.14 The main steps in the LPE segmentation algorithm.

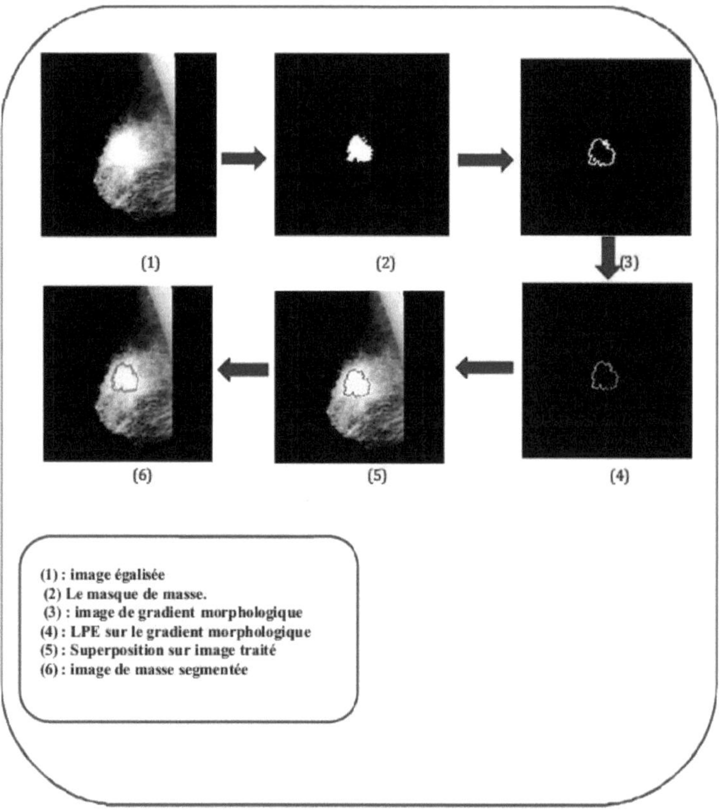

Figure 3.15 The different stages of water divide lines.

(1)   equalized image

(2)   The mass mask.

(3)   morphological gradient image

(4)   LPE on the morphological gradient

(5)   : Superimposition on processed image

(6)   segmented mass image

5.3.3 Segmentation by region (Regional growth)

Region growing is a simple method for segmenting breast lesions and is conceptually very easy and gives good results [41].However, this method has certain disadvantages:

> This is a semi-automatic method that requires user intervention for the choice of homogeneity criteria and germ initialization.

> Poor sprout selection or a poor choice of homogeneity measurement criteria can lead to over- or under-segmentation.

> Long calculation times.

We have developed an algorithm for the detection of breast masses based on region growth illustrated in the following figure:

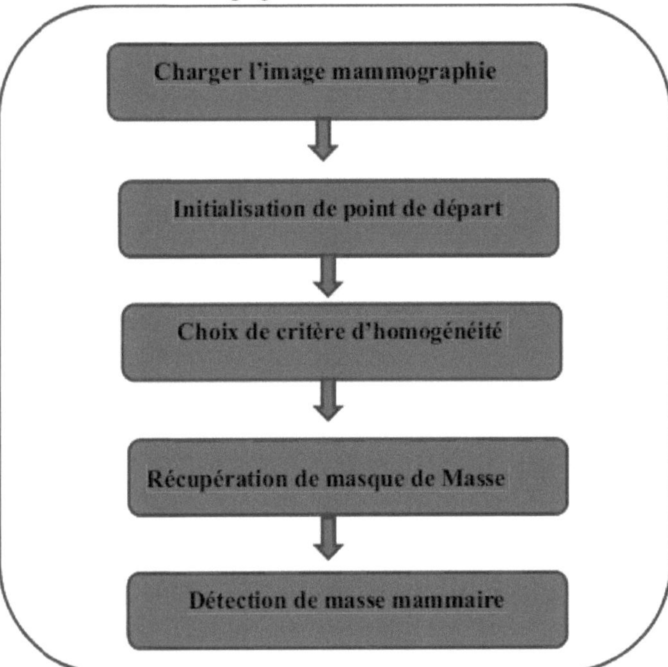

Figure 3.16: The main steps in the region-growth algorithm for detecting breast lumps.

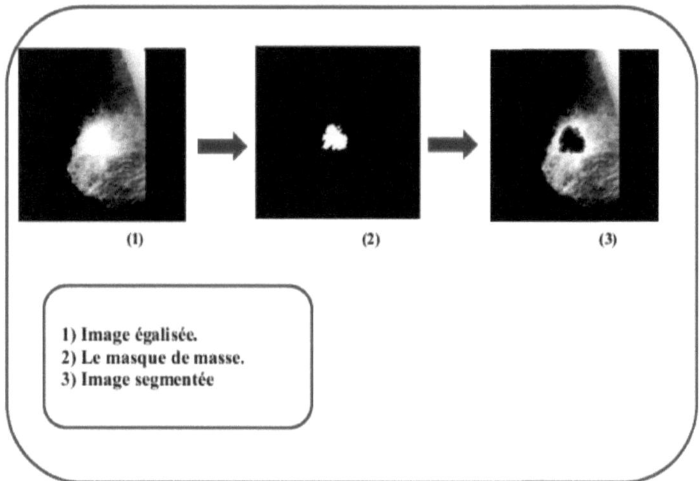

Figure 3.17 The different stages in region growth.

5.3.4 Unsupervised classification methods

These techniques are used when the identity of the classes is not known. This results from a lack of information about the population to be studied. Classification algorithms, consisting of several iterations, can be used to create groupings of individuals with similar characteristics. Unsupervised classification, known as automatic classification or clustering, consists of determining the different classes naturally, without any prior knowledge. In this case, the aim is to identify a structure in the images in the database based on their content. The images are assigned to the various classes estimated according to two essential criteria: the high degree of homogeneity of each class and good separation between the classes.

❖Segmentation by K-means

Among unsupervised classification methods, the most commonly used and best-known, due to its simplicity of implementation, is the K-means algorithm. This is the K-means algorithm, also known as the dynamic clustering algorithm. The algorithm works by specifying the number K of expected clusters (K is set by the user). It calculates the intra-class distance and refixes the class centres according to the distance values.

K-means is an iterative algorithm that minimises the sum of the distances between each object and the centroid of its cluster. The disadvantages of this method are, firstly, the need to fix the number of classes before starting the classification. Secondly, this method is very sensitive to the initial distribution of the data. Finally, this method assumes that the classes follow reduced normal distributions, in other words, with the same importance in all directions in space, which is not always the case.

To improve the K-means algorithm, follow these steps:

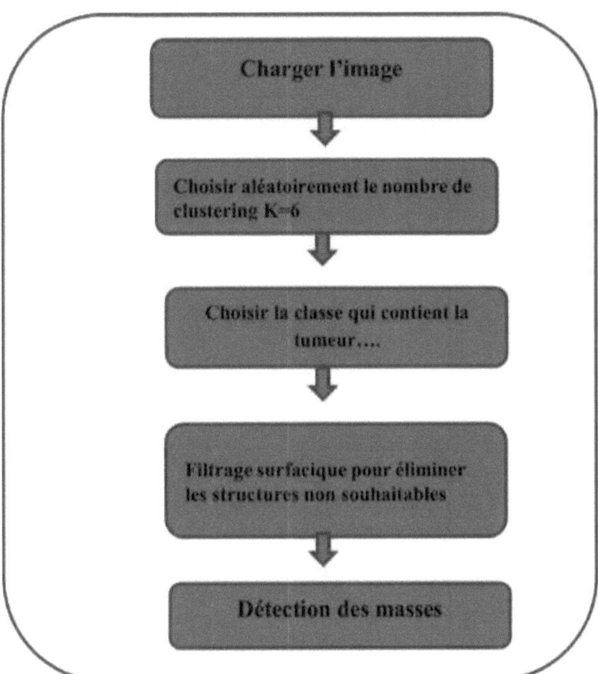

Figure 3.18 The main steps in the K-means algorithm.

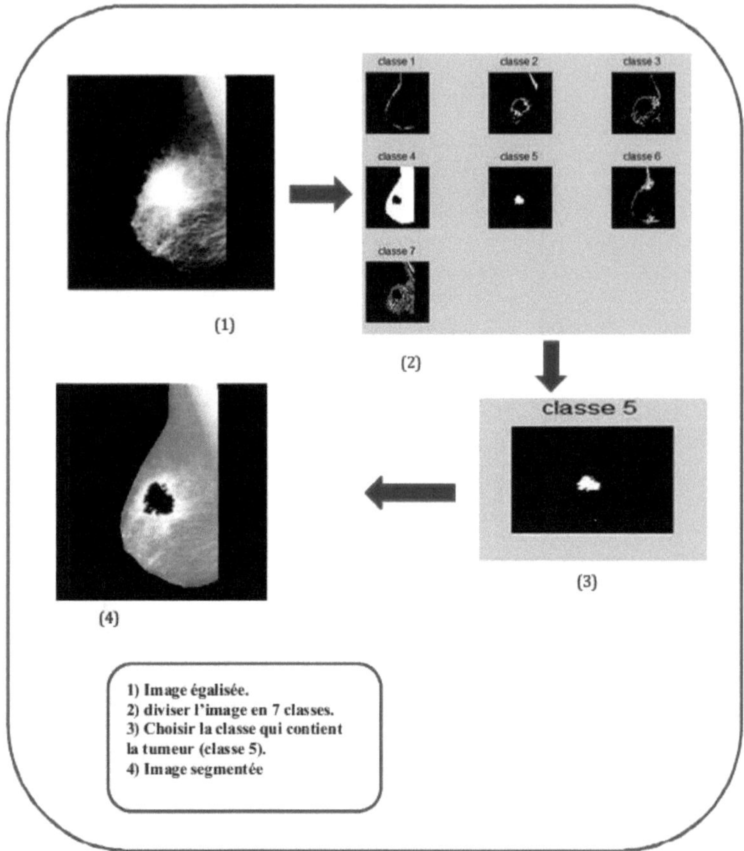

1)   Equalised image.
2)   divide the image into 7 classes.
3)   Choose the class containing the tumour (class 5).
4)   Segmented image

Figure 3.19 The different stages of the K-means approach.

6   *Results and discussion*

The pre-processing stage (mammary gland extraction, filtering and contrast enhancement) plays an important role in improving the results of breast lesion segmentation, especially in cases where the breast is dense or hyperdense, as detection is difficult even for the radiologist, whereas detection is easy where the breast density is low.

7   *Comparison of the three approaches :*

7.1 *Qualitative comparison :*

From the previous results we can see that segmentation by the three methods gives good results. In our case, however, we obtained good localization of the tumour (disease) using LPE segmentation, better than k-means and region growth.

7.2 Quantitative comparison :

Quantitative comparison is also an important comparison. We can calculate the ratio of the intersection (the number of common pixels) to the union (all the pixels in two images) to see which segmentation method is best.

> Good result the ratio is close to > Less good the ratio is close to

ApproachReportResults

LPE	0.0769	Good results
region growth	0.4003	Worst result
k-means	0.4801	Worst result

Table 2 Comparison of ratios between segmentation approaches

7.3 Discussion on Runtime

The difference between these segmentation approaches is the execution time, which varies for each of these three approaches.

The following table shows the execution time of each approach for different images:

Method mdb028 mdb184 mdb025 mdb081 mdb015 mdb134 mdb202

Method	mdb028	mdb184	mdb025	mdb081	mdb015	mdb134	mdb202
LPE	2,2639982	2,3433716	3,2085278	2,789609	2,692549	2,946026	2,660500
Regional growth	3,3221228	4,4312442	4,1425262	7,480537	3,680592	2,993379	2,619339
K-means	24,887732	29,832933	21,971981	22,01368	23,41433	15,62139	17,06345

Table 3 Comparison of execution times between segmentation approaches.

We have seen that the watershed approach is a powerful tool for segmenting breast masses, as it gives interesting results with a low computation time compared with other segmentation approaches.

8 Extraction of mammography characteristics

Once the mammogram has been segmented, the next step is to extract the features that describe the image regions, along with a few notions and definitions about classification.

8.1 Proposed approach

In order to detect breast masses in an "optimal" way, we will take advantage of the dynamic programming principle concerning optimality stated by the mathematician Richard Bellman: "Any optimal policy is composed of optimal sub-policies" [29]. In other words, any optimal solution is itself based on sub-problems solved locally in an optimal way.

In practical terms, this means that we can deduce the optimal solution to our problem by combining the optimal solutions of a series of sub-problems. The solutions of the problems are studied "from the bottom up", i.e. we calculate the solutions of the smallest sub-problems and then gradually deduce the solutions of the whole.

In our case, our big problem is made up of four sub-problems:

1) Better pre-treatment
2) Best segmentation approach
3) Best descriptor
4) Best classifier

In this thesis we have concentrated on the first three problems, and to solve them we have studied and implemented several algorithms for pre-processing as well as for segmentation. The following figure shows the process and the algorithms used.

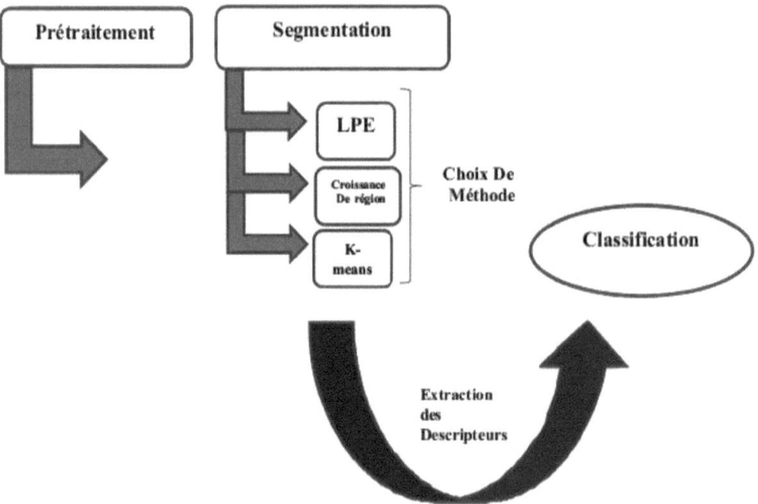

Figure3.20: Methodology of our work

8.2 *Shape descriptors in mammography (geometric)*

The choice of attributes to characterise a region is a difficult problem that requires all the experience of the image processor. The choice depends on the image to be processed and the problem to be solved. From the results of the segmentation applied to the images, we obtain a map of homogeneous regions where the pixels in each region carry a single value characterising the region [42].

We have chosen the following parameters as descriptors:

8.2.1 *The surface*

One of the most common shape descriptors is the mass area, which is calculated from the number of pixels contained in a lesion.

Surface $=\Sigma\Sigma b$ (i, j). (3.5)

8.2.2 *Perimeter*

The calculation of the perimeter of the mass noted P is also commonly used in the field of breast cancer diagnosis. It refers to the number of pixels in the contour.

Perimeter $= \Sigma c$ (i, j). (3.6)

8.2.3 Circularity

$$C = 4\pi S / P^2 \quad (3.7)$$

Where P is the perimeter of the object and S is the area in pixels.

Circularity represents the way in which a shape is similar to a circle; it tends towards 1 for perfectly round shapes and is lower the more irregular the shape [43].

8.2.4 Compactness

$$\text{Compactness} = P^2 / S. \quad (3.8)$$

Where P is the perimeter of the object and A is the area in pixels. This compactness value is used to distinguish an irregular shape from a simple shape, as it gives the irregular shape a higher value.

8.2.5 Centre of gravity

Since the centre of gravity C (xi, yi) of an object is frequently used to define shape descriptors, we first define it. This measure is closely related to the shape of the object, so the coordinates (xi, yi) of the centre of gravity are defined as follows:

$$Ci = \Sigma\, xi / n \quad (3.9)$$

$$Cj = \Sigma\, yi / n$$

With n: number of pixels (area).

After segmenting the different objects in the image and extracting these characteristics, we can say that this operation enables classification [42].

8.2.6 Eccentricity

Scalar, which defines the eccentricity of the ellipse, it is easy to define (based on its major and minor axes) the enclosing box with the same orientation as the object under consideration. The value is between 0 and 1. (0 and 1 are degenerate cases, an ellipse whose eccentricity is 0 is in fact a circle, whereas an ellipse whose eccentricity is 1 is a straight line segment). This property is only supported for input 2-D label matrices.

Example of calculation of the previous descriptors:

Abbreviations :

P=perimeter S=surface C= circularity	E=eccentricity Gx, Gy=centre of gravity Com=compactness	LPE=water sharing line RG=region growth KM=K_Means

The images	mdb028			mdb 184			mdb 134			mdb 015		
Methods	LPE	RG	KM	LPE	RG	KM	LPE	RG	KM	LPE	RG	KM
P	356	422	403	558	640	643	254	283	234	293	326	280
S	7574	7569	8336	17046	16937	19929	3754	3743	3239	5014	5724	4198
C	0.75	0.53	0.64	0.69	0.52	0.61	0.73	0.59	0.74	0.73	0.68	0.67
Com	16.72	22.52	20.29	18.27	25.65	20.75	17.24	20.49	16.54	16.59	18.03	17.51
E	0.52	0.58	0.47	0.70	0.68	0.64	0.47	0.45	0.61	0.81	0.78	0.77
Gx	708	742	706	397	410	398	292	313	297	160	168	160
Gy	344	361	338	357	369	351	470	502	468	601	629	603

Table 3.4: Calculation of geometric descriptors.

8.3 Texture descriptors in mammography

Various methods of extracting texture characteristics can be applied to the search for areas in a mammogram. One of these methods is the co-occurrence matrix. Features based on co-occurrence matrices (SGLD Spatial Gray Level Dependency Matrices): this is a statistical method that consists of constructing co-occurrence matrices (SGLD) to represent the relationships between pixels in an image. The matrix represents the joint probability of two grey levels i, j being in a given spatial relationship. This relationship is defined in terms of the distance and angle between these two pixels. The angle is used to evaluate the texture direction and the application of several distance values can give a meaningful description of the size of the texture periodicity [42]. Many features can be extracted from these matrices, some of which are listed below:

8.3.1 Contrast

Returns a measure of the contrast intensity between a pixel and its neighbour in the whole image, defined by the relation :

$$\Sigma i, j \; (i - j) \; 2 \; p \; (i, j) \quad (3.10)$$

8.3.2 Correlation

This parameter is used to determine whether certain columns of the matrix are equal, i.e. whether there are linear dependencies in the image. It measures the linear dependency of the grey levels in the image. Correlation is not correlated with either energy or entropy. It has an important value if the columns and rows of the matrix are uniform.

$$\Sigma \; (i-\mu i) \; (j-\mu j) \; p \; (i, j) \; / \; \sigma i \sigma j. \quad (3.11)$$

8.3.3 Energy

Energy measures the homogeneity of the image. The lower this value, the less uniform the image, and it is defined by the relationship :

$$\Sigma \; i, \; (i, j) \; 2 \quad \textbf{(3.12)}$$

8.3.4 Homogeneity

Returns a value that measures the proximity of the distribution of elements in the GLCM to the GLCM diagonal, defined by the relation :

$$\Sigma \; P \; (i, j) \; / \; i, j \; 1+|i-j| \quad (3.13)$$

9   Classification

Classification is considered to be the final stage in a computer-aided diagnosis (CADx) system. It uses the description result (which in turn uses the segmentation result) to decide on the pathological nature of the mass.

The notion of classification means assigning a label to samples in a database using a certain number of characteristics. These characteristics must, of course, be able to identify each sample. In image processing, ^sample can refer to a pixel, an area in the image, an object represented in the image or the image itself. Depending on the application, the aim of classification is either to :

> classify image pixels into different zones. In this case, the classification problem amounts to a problem of segmenting images into different objects. For example, the different zones of a mammographic image can be classified as lesion or non-lesion.

> classify the image or the objects in the image according to different categories. Examples include

> classify masses in mammographic images as malignant or benign.

There are two types of classification:

> Supervised classification: the classes are known in advance and generally have an associated semantics

> Unsupervised classification: the classes are based on the structure of the objects, the semantics associated with the classes are more difficult to determine [42].

10 Development environment

10.1 MATLAB mammography programming language :

MATLAB is short for *Matrix LABoratory*. Originally written in Fortran by *C. Moler*, MATLAB was intended to facilitate access to matrix software. We will come back to this point, which is a fundamental element of the MATLAB language: most of the functions defined in MATLAB are for matrix quantities, and by extension, for tabulated data.

MATLAB also includes a set of domain-specific tools called Toolboxes. Essential for most users, Toolboxes are collections of functions that extend the MATLAB environment to solve specific classes of problems. The areas covered are very varied and include signal and image processing, automatic control, system identification, neural networks, fuzzy logic, structure calculation, statistics, etc.

Image Processing Toolbox provides a complete set of standard reference algorithms, functions and applications for image processing, analysis, visualisation and algorithm development. You can perform a wide range of operations, including image analysis, image segmentation, image enhancement, noise removal, geometric transformations and image registration. Image Processing Toolbox supports a diverse set of image, visualization functions and applications that allow you to explore images and videos, examine an area of pixels, adjust contrast and colour, create contours or histograms, and manipulate regions of interest (ROIs). The toolbox supports development workflows for processing, displaying and exploring large images.

10.2 The application's main interfaces

In this section, we present the software that carries out the segmentation methods and their application to mammography images. An interface that can be made available to users with all possible freedom, taking advantage of the capacity of programming languages such as MATLAB. Home interface

Our application consists of a welcome window containing information about the project and the **Enter** button for accessing the application.

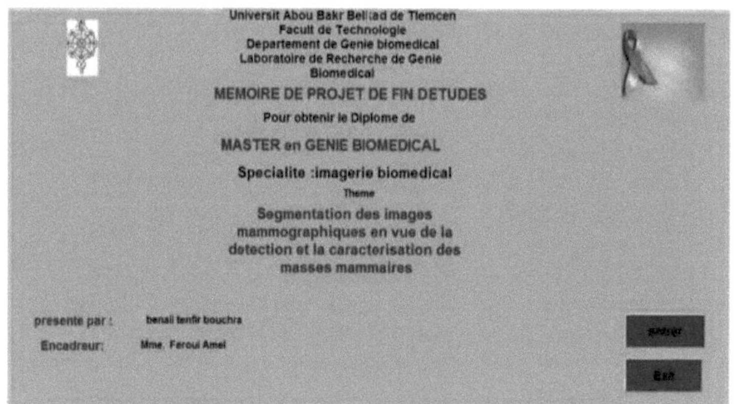

Figure 4. 21: Home interface

When the **Enter** button is pressed from the Home screen, the following interface appears, containing buttons that allow us to choose our algorithms

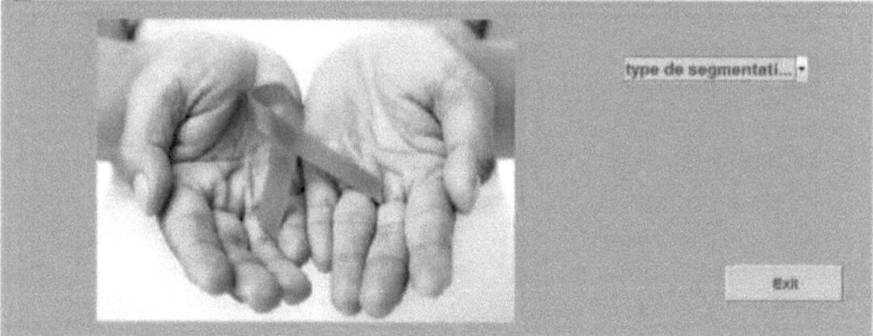

Figure 4. 22: Home interface 2

10.4 Pre-processing interface :

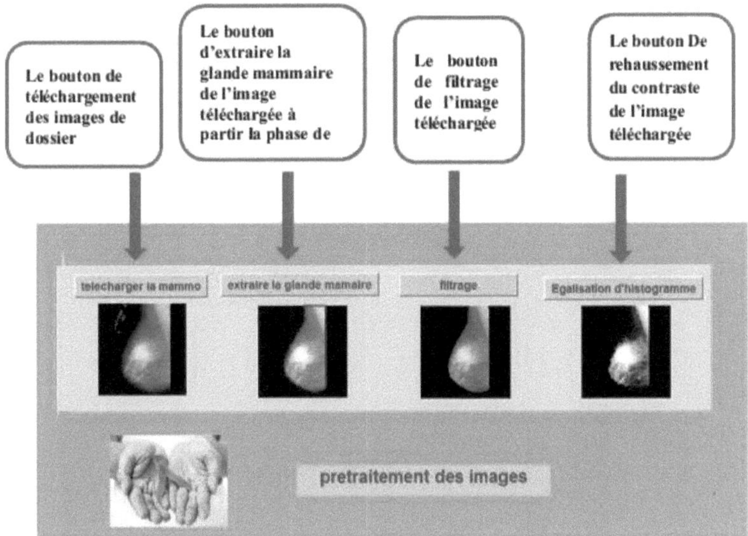

Figure 4. 23 : Pre-processing interface

10.5 Segmentation interface

This is the application's main interface and is made up of 3 interfaces (a) , (b) , (c).

❖ **Interfaces (a)**

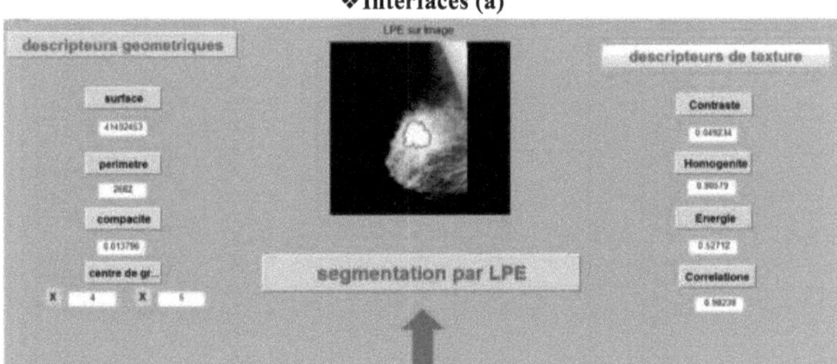

The end of the image segmentation downloaded by the watershed lines
Figure 4. 24 : Interface (a)

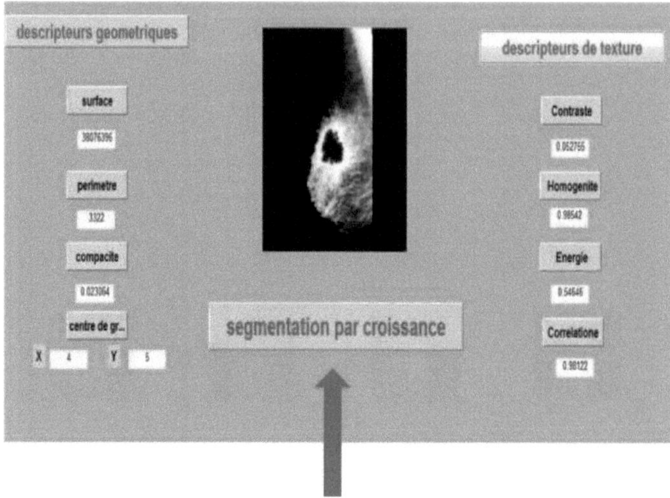

The segmentation button of the image downloaded by the Growth region interface (b).

Figure 4. 25 : Interface (b)

❖ **Interfaces (c)**

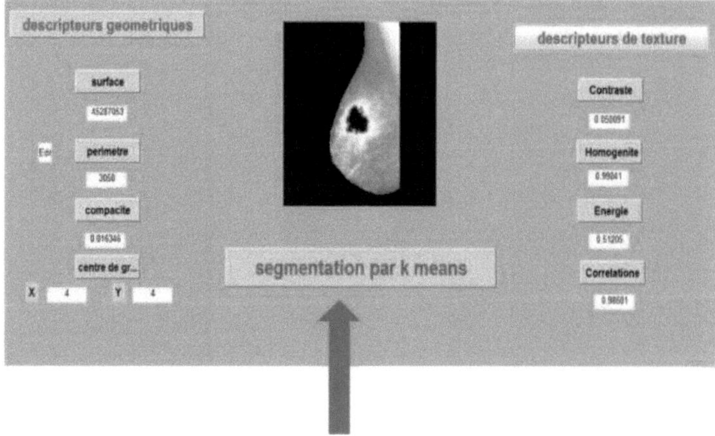

The image segmentation button Downloaded using the K-meansv interface (c).

Figure 4. 26 : Interface (c)

11 Conclusion

In this chapter, we have presented some image processing tools for the pre-processing of mammographic images, the aim of which is to eliminate undesirable structures in order to facilitate the segmentation of opacities, which are the focus of this thesis.

In the 1st part of this work, we presented an algorithm based on a few morphological operators and contrast enhancement with the aim of extracting the mammary gland with a cleaned background (removal of mammography artefacts). To improve segmentation algorithms.

In the second part, we applied the various segmentation algorithms to all the images processed. The algorithms proposed in this chapter give excellent results for mammograms. Then, a comparative study between the results of these methods allows us to conclude that the marker-controlled watershed line is a powerful tool for segmenting breast opacities with a small computation time but it is sensitive to noise, the other region growth method gives efficient results provided a good criterion term is chosen and the last K means method takes a powerful time with satisfactory results.

It seems impossible to design an algorithm that gives good results for all images, which proves that human interaction is still necessary.

In the third part, we presented our working method, which consisted of extracting shape and texture attributes encoded in greyscale,

Matlab is a powerful image-processing tool, which made it easier for us to exploit and process the mammographic masses.

12 General conclusion and outlook

In this work, we are interested in the study of medical imaging as an aid to the diagnosis of breast cancer, in particular the description of breast masses. Statistics confirm that breast cancer represents a major threat to a woman's life. However, such a threat can only be managed by prompt treatment of the disease to maximise the chances of survival. The aim is to use the results of the various segmentation approaches to :

> Early detection of breast cancer.

> Reducing radiologist error

> Extraction of quantitative parameters to determine the nature of lesions, thereby reducing the number of unnecessary biopsies.

> Correct classification of lesions.

In this project, we apply a pre-processing phase on the MIAS database images with the MATLAB language in order to Recover the breast area with a cleaned background, then we use the segmentation approaches of LPE and region growth and K-means, with each method we extract shape characteristics (surface, perimeter, compactness...) and texture attributes (energy, homogeneity ....) calculated on the co-occurrence matrix. In order to elaborate the classification part successfully.

We note that the different segmentation methods give convergent results and don't have a big difference between them in terms of contour, but in terms of execution time the k-means is very expensive.

The results of this study were satisfactory in the light of the results presented in the literature and confirmed by radiologists. The results of this study are encouraging. However, we found certain problems, such as the lack of real mammography images and the absence of the support from doctors and radiologists that is needed in our work.

> **Prospects and possible follow-up to this work...**

This dissertation has given rise to a number of perspectives, which we summarise as follows A few lines:

1. There is a strong link between the concept of segmentation and classification: once the relevant parameters have been extracted, classification can be envisaged to identify a benign or malignant anomaly.

2. A logical extension of this approach is system automation.

Of course, this list is by no means exhaustive, and a good number of additional extensions can certainly be imagined...

Bibliography

[1] J. Brettes, C. Mathelin, B. Gairard, J. Bellocq. Cancer du sein. Paris: Elsevier Masson, 2007. 358 p. ISBN: 978-2-294-01813-8.

[2] http: //sante-medecine.journaldesfemmes.com/contents/132-breast-cancer-symptoms-and-treatment

[3] Les maladies du sein http: //www.e-cancer.fr/Patients-et-proches/Les-cancers/Cancer-dusein/Les-maladies-du-sein, visit on 12/2019.

[4] BREAST CANCER, WHAT IS IT   , http : //www.soscancerdusein.org/soscancer-du-sein-cancer-du-sein-32.html, visited 12/2015.

[5] http://www.ass.nc/themes/cancer-du-sein/moyens-de-depistage

[6] Imaging medical http://www.doctissimo.fr/html/sante/imagerie/imagerie_sommaire.htm#echographie, visited in November 2019.

[7] Imen cheikhrouhou Esp kachouri. "Description et classification des masses mammaires pour le diagnostic du cancer du sein", thesis for the title of doctor at the University of Evry-Val d'Essonne.

[8] S. H. Kobrunner, I. Schreer, R. Bassler, M. Dickhaut. Diagnostic breast imaging Mammography, ultrasound, MRI, interventional techniques.

[10] H. Chekkaf, I. Touil, Mass segmentation in Mammographic images, Thesis for the Master of Science degree in Computer Science, 2019.

[11] P. Haehnel. Mammography - 83 radiodiagnostic exercises for students and practitioners. Paris: Vigot, 1996. 137p. Radiodiagnostic exercises. ISBN: 2-7114- 1049.

[12] CJ. VYBORNY 'Can computers help radiologists read mammograms ?

[13] Raffi ENFICIAUD, "Algorithmes multidimensionnels et multi spectraux en Morphologie Mathématique : Approche par méta-programmation", Thesis to obtain the grade de Docteur de l'ecole des Mines de Paris Spécialité " Morphologie Mathématique " on 26 February 2019.

[14] Giovanni palma, "automatic detection of opacities in digital breast tomosynthesis", february 23,2019.

[15] CHIKH Mohammed Tahar, "Amélioration des images par un modèle de réseau de neurones (Comparaison avec les filtres de base)", Memoire de fin d'etudes pour l'obtention du diplôme de Master en Informatique 2011.

[16] K. Chakib, Compression des images fixes par les approximations fractales Basée, Mémoire de fin d'études, 1999.

[17] I. Hadjidj, Approche Morphologique pour la Segmentation d'Images Médicales, Dissertation presented to the University of Tlemcen for the award of the Diplôme de Magister en Électronique Biomédicale, 2011.

[18] J. P. Cocquerez, S. Philipp, "Image analysis: filtering and segmentation", Masson, Paris, 1995.

[19] Priyanka, Balwinder Singh, "A review on brain tumor detection using segmentation".

[20] Lecoeur, C.Barillot, "Segmentation d'images cerebrales" : Etat de l'art Rapport de recherche, Institut INI, version révisée en 2019.

[21] KESSOUR Islam and TALI Imane, "Simulation des contours actifs par les colonies de fourmis", Pour l'obtention du diplôme d'Ingenieur d'Etat en Informatique 2019.

[22] L.S.A. Bins, L. M. G. Foncseca, G.J. Erthal and F. M. Ii, "Satellite imagery segmentation: to region growing approach", in 8 Brazilian Symposium Remote Sensing, pp.

677-680, 1996.

[23] U. C. Benz, P. Hofmann, G. Willhauck, I. Lingenfelder, M. Heynen, "Multi resolution, object-oriented fuzzy analysis of remote sensing data for GIS-ready information". ISPRS Journal of Photo grammetry & Remote Sensing, 58(3-4), pp.239-258, 2004.

[24] Baillie, J.C. "Cours de Segmentation Module D9 : traitement d'images et vision Artificielle".

[25] Ouarda ASSAS, "Classification floue des images", DOCTORAT EN SCIENCES Université de Batna 2013.

[26] S. L. Horowitz, T. Pavlidis, "Picture segmentation by tree transversal algorithm". J. ACM, Vol. 32, 2, pp. 368 G 388, 1976.

[27] R. C. Gonzalez and R. E. Woods, "Digital Image Processing". 2ed, Prentice Hall.

[28] N. Otsu, "A threshold selection method from grey-level histograms", IEEE transactions On systems, man, and cybernetics, vol. smc-9, no.1, January 1979, pp. 62-66.

[29] J. Mohanalin, M. Beenamol, "A new wavelet algorithm to enhance and detect

[30] L. Li, W. Qian, L. P. Clarke, R. A. Clark and J. A. Thomas, "Improving mass detection By adaptive and multiscale processing in digitized mammograms", Proc. SPIE, vol. 3661, pp. 490-498.

[31] The mini-MIAS database of mammograms, http://peipa.essex.ac.uk/info/mias

[32] khotanlou, "Segmentation 3D de tumeurs et de structures internes du cerveau en IRM, These de doctorat, l'ecole nationale superieure des telecommunications.

[33] Jean Jaques Rousselle. Active contours, segmentation method. Application a L'imagerie medicale. These Universite Fracois Rabelais de Tours.

[34] J.M. Rendon Mancha, "Régions Actives Morphologiques : Application à la Vision par Ordinateur", Doctoral thesis, Université René Descartes - Paris V.

[35] Ismahen HADJIJ. "Analyse des Images Mammographiques pour l'Aide à la Détection du Cancer du Sein", dissertation to obtain the degree of DOCTEUR EN SCIENCES EN ÉLECTRONIQUE BIOMÉDICALE.

[36] http: //peipa.essex.ac.uk/info/mias.html, visited January 2019.

[37] L. Belkhodja, N. Benamrane. Approche d'extraction de la région globale d'intérêt et suppression des artefacts radio pâques dans une image mammographique, Laboratoire d'Imagerie Vision Artificielle et Robotique Médicale Département d'Informatique Faculté des Sciences. IMAGE'09 Biskra.

[38] K. Chakib, Compression des images fixes par les approximations fractales Basée, Mémoire de fin d'études.

[39] CHIKH Mohammed Tahar, "Amélioration des images par un modèle de réseau de neurones (Comparaison avec les filtres de base)", Memoire de fin d'etudes pour l'obtention du diplôme de Master en Informatique 2011.

[40] Jean-Jacques ROUSSELLE, "Contours actifs, une méthode de segmentation application à l'imagerie médicale", Thesis to obtain the degree of Doctor in Computer Science from the University of Tours and defended by: 9/07/2003 Université François Rabelais de Tours.

[41] KESSOUR Islam and TALI Imane, "Simulation des contours actifs par les colonies de fourmis", Pour l'obtention du diplôme d'Ingenieur d'Etat en Informatique 2011.

[42] Imen cheikhrouhou Esp kachouri (defended 27 June 2012). "Description et classification des masses mammaires pour le diagnostic du cancer du sein", thesis for the title of doctor at the University of Evry- Val d'Essonne.

[43] Rachida LAKHDARI. (2011). "La détection des micros calcifications dans l'image Mammographie ", Mémoire présenté à l'Univenté à l'Univer

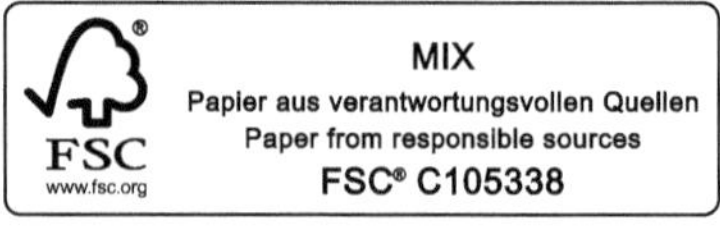

Printed by Books on Demand GmbH, Norderstedt / Germany